Rethinking Fat Loss

7 Must Know Mental Secrets to Success

Diana R. Chaloux - LaCerte

Table of Contents

DEDICATION

To our Hitch Fit clients worldwide who have allowed us to be a part of their transformation journey. Thank you for being a part of the mission to create a healthier world, one person at a time! Thank you to God for the blessing of living a purpose filled life. Thank you to my husband Micah for non-stop support and love!

Introduction

You've tried it all. Every diet, every new workout program.

It seems like NOTHING WORKS. At least not for the long term.

I get it. I was once in your shoes.

It's frustrating.

You want to live in a body that serves you well, and you find yourself stuck in one that doesn't.

You want to look in the mirror and be happy with how you look and feel, but you don't.

You're ready for a change.

Maybe, just like I did, you've reached a point where you say, enough is enough. There are fit and healthy people in this world, and you're ready to become one of them.

You've got a goal, and this time you're going to achieve it.

Is this you?

If you see transformation photos and you long to be one of those success stories. If you want to know what it feels like to live in a body that you love, have a healthy body fat, "tone up" or change your eating habits in a healthy way, then I wrote this book for you.

I am going to share the secrets you need to know, and action steps that you need to take BEFORE, DURING and AFTER your fitness journey.

Whether you decide you would like to work with me (or my husband Micah) as your coach, or if you go a different route, you will be able to use the valuable information in this book to help you mentally be prepared for success.

I'd like to teach you the secrets for LONG TERM success and not just a quick fix fast weight loss (meaning lose weight and then gain it right back).

In *"Rethinking Fat Loss"* I will discuss the top 7 mental secrets that I consider to be the keys to not just losing body fat, but creating a healthy body that you can live in for life.

If you read this book and have questions for me, or would like to share about your personal story and see how Micah and I could help, please feel free to contact us, or connect with us via social media. We are easily accessible. Helping people succeed is what we thrive on, so we would love to hear from you!

My "WHY":

Before we get started, I'll give you a little background on WHY this topic of transformation is so near and dear to my heart.

The things I'm sharing with you in this book are what I've had to learn first-hand in order to not just lose 50 pounds, but to keep it off (as of now it has been 14 years!). If I hadn't learned the secrets I'm sharing, there's no way I would have kept the weight off. I would have continued the yo-yo for years.

The weight gain crept up on me. I was active all through my childhood. I engaged in sports on a regular basis when I was in my youth. Eating whatever I wanted didn't lead to weight gain at that time.

In my mid-20's I started gaining little by little. I noticed my clothes didn't fit as well, I didn't have the energy that I wanted, I wasn't comfortable in my own skin. But rather than face the problem, I just kept buying new clothes and making excuses for myself.

I worked out all the time, but my eating habits were terrible, though I refused to admit that to myself. Drinking alcohol on a regular basis and engaging in compulsive over eating and binge eating behaviors every night, was wreaking havoc on my body and my health.

And guess what. All through this, I was a personal trainer! It's true!

I began personal training in 2002. I learned all about the exercise side of things and taking people through workouts. But learning how to eat to work in conjunction with training (to get your body to do what you want it to!) was not something that was taught, and not something I understood.

I have to apologize to the clients who I worked with early on, who came to me for anything other than gaining strength. If their goal was weight loss, then I couldn't help them. I simply didn't know what to tell them to do.

I cringe at some of the terrible advice that I gave people in those days. I had no idea about what people should eat, how much they should eat and when they should eat it in order to achieve their fat loss goals. They were coming to a personal trainer for weight loss, and at that time, I simply wasn't equipped with the knowledge I needed to help them achieve that goal.

I worked as a fitness director for Norwegian Cruise Lines for a year, from 2004 – 2005. It was the dream job! Travel and fitness all rolled into one! I was ecstatic to be on this adventure, but soon found myself lonely.

My binge eating behaviors became consistently worse, especially at night when I was alone in my cabin.

The scale went up… and up… and up. Even though, as the fitness director, I was working out all day long!

I stepped on the scale one day. It soared up over 175 pounds (which was the most I had ever weighed). I jumped off. I got a lump in my throat and a knot in my belly. What was I doing to myself? This was about 30 - 35 pounds more than I weighed when I arrived on the ship. It had been less than a year.

I felt out of control in that moment. I knew that my binge eating behaviors were the reason for the gain, but I didn't know how to stop them. It was scary to think that I didn't have the self-control to make a different choice for myself.

I didn't change right away. I stayed on the ship for several more months, and finally in February 2005, my ship life was over.

When my little sister, Maria, saw me for the first time (in over a year) her jaw dropped. She didn't say anything. She didn't want to hurt my feelings. But I could see the shock at my weight gain on her face. My family loves me no matter what size I am, but I know that it was shocking to see that I had let my health decline in this way.

Procrastination is a killer. But I did it anyways.

I did lose about 10 pound within a few weeks of getting off the ship, simply because I wasn't going to the crew bar every night, and didn't have all the highly caloric foods right at my fingertips. But I was still binge eating at night, when everyone else had gone to bed.

I moved to San Antonio, TX in spring of 2005 to live with my older sister, Linda. I was hired as a personal trainer at a local gym. I made some friends from the gym, but the normal became going out to bars and clubs on the weekends. Even though I was telling my clients to make healthy choices, I wasn't doing it myself.

I felt like a fraud.

Finally on July 5, 2005 I had my "aha" moment that changed the trajectory of my life for good.

After partying on the 4th of July, drinking beer and even going to McDonalds for a caramel sundae, I came into work feeling bloated and disgusted with myself. How on earth could I come in here and pretend I was a healthy person when this was my behavior?

A fellow trainer, Bill, was in the gym that morning. He greeted me with a smile and said, "Hey, I saw on your bio that you want to do figure competitions? What are you waiting for?"

I froze for a second. I didn't have an answer.

Yes, this had been a dream of mine for YEARS. I had pictures of fitness women from *Oxygen* magazine, that I admired, plastered all over my walls as motivation. Yet, that had not done the trick to actually get me to DO what I needed to do to get the result I wanted to achieve.

My mind wasn't right yet.

But in this instant. That question triggered the change in my mind that I needed. It triggered me from just "wanting" my goal, to wanting it enough to actually take action towards it.

I didn't wait until Monday, I didn't procrastinate for a moment longer. I changed, THAT DAY.

I changed my eating habits (not perfectly just yet, I had a LOT of learning to do!). I looked for a show that was far enough out that I would have time to prepare for it. But I wanted a deadline that would motivate me.

I took before pictures so I could acknowledge exactly where I was, and then set my sites on where I wanted to go.

And then I did it.

I changed MY MIND.

I didn't make excuses anymore. I didn't look back. I didn't tell myself that I was a "victim" for not getting to eat this that or the other thing (trust me, I had eaten and drank enough junk to last a lifetime!). I just did it. One day at a time, one choice at a time.

Seeing progress was motivating. Seeing my body change little by little is what kept me persevering.

It didn't happen fast, it didn't happen overnight. But over the course of about 5 months I shed nearly 50 pounds of body fat and was ready to step on stage at my very first show!

The best part about this transformation wasn't winning the show (which I did!!), it was realizing that my mindset had changed enough that the emotional eating and compulsive over eating habits no longer had control over me.

The discipline of training and focusing on this goal had UNLEASHED me from the bondage of those limiting behaviors.

I was finally FREE. I felt FREE.

I was free of turning to food for emotional support (which it didn't provide to begin with). I was free from living in a body that I didn't like how it looked and that felt puffy and bloated. I was free from the feeling that I was a fraud for talking about a healthy lifestyle and not living it. It was all freedom, and it felt GOOD.

The reason I'm so passionate about helping people transform is because I've been there myself. I've had to walk the walk that I'm teaching people. I've taken every step personally, and I know how hard it can be, but I also know how worth it, it is, when you get to the other side.

I've lived on both sides, in a body that I didn't feel well in, and in a body that I love living in and that gives me the freedom to enjoy my life to the fullest.

I know what it's like to have a weak mindset that left me stuck, and I know what it feels like to intentionally shift my mental attitude and strengthen my thoughts so that they work for me and not against me.

I've had to dig deep and do the work to find out why I was making poor choices to begin with. I had to face my fears and insecurities, I had to confront pain from the past so that it no longer held me captive.

I changed my mind. I made new choices. That led to my body physically changing too!

I choose healthy. I choose fit. I choose strong. I choose it because it's worth it.

This is why, when I met the love of my life, my husband Micah, in 2008, we decided to start Hitch Fit, and help people transform their minds and their lives, the same way I had transformed mine.

Now, of course, not everyone wants to do a competition. That was just me. It's not the right path for everyone, it was what motivated me to make the changes that I needed to.

But many people, just like you if you're reading this book, want to change. And maybe it's because of something external, like how you look on the outside, but even more, it's about the internal.

Maybe it's your health. Not taking care of your body can lead to debilitating diseases. It can make it so you can't do the things that you want to do physically (like go on a hike or ride a bike, or play with the kids). It can give you low self-esteem or confidence which can impact your relationships with others, relationship with your spouse (lack of intimacy because you don't feel good about your body) and even job performance.

It can impact the energy that you feel through the day, leaving you lethargic and tired.

We have a lot of transformation success stories at Hitch Fit. Thousands of before and after photos of clients that we've worked with either online or at our gyms in Kansas City. But what Micah and I have discovered is that the external transformation is just the icing on the cake. It's all the changes that have happened on the inside that have truly transformed a person's life.

I'd recommend grabbing a journal as you read through this

book. Take your time reflecting on the questions asked, write out your thoughts, ideas, realizations and responses as you go through this process.

Let's do this. I know that you can. I'm excited to see you take these first steps towards the healthiest and best version of you.

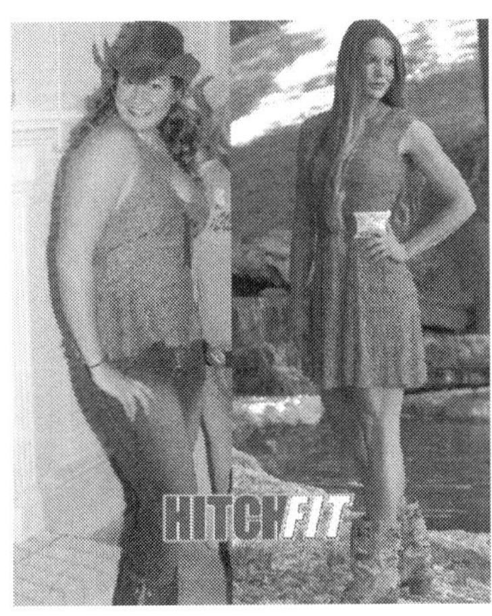

Check out MY weight loss story and before and after photos here: https://hitchfit.com/about-hitch-fit/diana-chaloux-lacerte-top-fitness-model/

Hear about my battle with Emotional Eating and how I overcame it here: https://hitchfit.com/success-stories/lose-weight-stories/my-weight-loss-journey-hitch-fit-owner-shares-emotional-truth/

Chapter 1.

MIND SHIFTS:

Change Your Perception

Are you ready to change something in your life?

I'm assuming the answer is YES!

I'll take that a step further and guess that one of the changes you're hoping for has to do with your physical fitness and health. (This is a book about fat loss after all!).

If that's the case, there is a FIRST step that you have to take.

You must take note of, and make necessary shifts to your mind and thought processes.

Henry Ford nailed it on the head when he said "Whether you think you can or you think you can't, you're right."

This is so true! You can achieve what your mind believes. But the first step to self-sabotage is allowing negative thoughts to pervade your mind and have an impact on your reality.

Too often, we don't even realize that these limiting beliefs are directing our choices and outcomes. It becomes a force of habit to list off all the reasons we "can't" do something, without even realizing that it simply isn't the truth.

How do you identify if you need a mental shift?

Action Step #1 – Pay attention to Self-Talk.

The first step is paying attention to your self-talk, and the chatter that goes through your mind.

You have the ability to notice your thoughts, think about your thoughts, and even change your thoughts.

There isn't a lot in this world that we have complete control over, but our thoughts are one thing that we can control and direct! It does take practice and it takes intentionality, but it can be done.

Your mind is constantly moving, thoughts go in and out all through the day. Have you ever stopped to really take notice of them?

What do you find yourself thinking about?

Are your thoughts predominantly negative or positive?

When situations occur that are beyond your control, do you see what the positive or the blessing could be? Or do you look at the negative side and dwell on it?

When you think about yourself, are your thoughts positive and uplifting or do you tear yourself down?

Every word out of your mouth, every action that you take, every belief you have about yourself, every story you have told yourself is true of you, every reaction or response you have, every feeling, every emotion, every choice, every perception of the world around you, began with a THOUGHT. YOUR thought.

Thoughts are the origin of everything you experience in your life.

Our mind controls our brains and our brains control our bodies. If we can change our thoughts, and re-wire our minds, we can literally change the outcomes in every other aspect of our lives. That's why we have to begin with what is happening in our minds.

Thoughts are things. I'm a huge fan of the research and books of Dr. Caroline Leaf.[1] If you're not familiar with Dr. Leaf, she has dedicated her life to researching the brain. She teaches how we can better understand our minds and how they either lead us in creating successful or unsuccessful lives.

She is a pioneer in the area of neuroplasticity – the study of how changes in thinking, change the brain and effect behavior.

A few key things to understand about our thought life:[2]

1. **Thoughts are THINGS.**
2. **Thinking creates thoughts that become actual protein matter in the brain.**
3. **We have power and authority to direct our thoughts.**
4. **We have free will and the ability to choose what we think about.**
5. **We can think about our thoughts.**

---

[1] Leaf, Caroline. *Switch on Your Brain: the Key to Peak Happiness, Thinking, and Health*. BakerBooks, a Division of Baker Publishing Group, 2015.

[2] Leaf, Caroline. *Switch on Your Brain: the Key to Peak Happiness, Thinking, and Health*. BakerBooks, a Division of Baker Publishing Group, 2015.

6. **We are capable of recognizing our thoughts and re-directing them.**
7. **Thoughts impact the actual structure of the brain.**
8. **Toxic thoughts can cause brain damage. Healthy thoughts can repair brain damage.**
9. **Thoughts impact our brain, which in turn impacts our body.**
10. **Intentionally removing toxic thought patterns and creating new healthy thought patterns IS possible.**

The ability to change your brain through your thoughts is not wishful thinking, it is scientifically based truth. Knowing this gives hope for what is possible if you will commit to the process of intentionally changing your thoughts.

One of the best ways to wrangle your thoughts is by journaling. Get yourself a new journal that suits you. Maybe one that has an inspirational quote on the cover. You can journal for just a few minutes or for hours. There's no right or wrong to it!

Let your thoughts pour out on paper, you'll easily be able to look back and see if they have a negative or positive vibe to them.

Don't try to edit your writing, just let the thoughts flow. If you jump from topic to topic, that is ok! This exercise of journaling will help you discover the thought areas that need improvement.

Journals are also great for giving you something to look back on over time. You'll be able to see the changes you have in thinking, and see how far you have come.

If you find that your thoughts are mostly positive, that you have a "CAN DO" attitude in most areas, then good for you,

you're off to a great start! You can take a look and see if there are any areas of life that you DO have a negative belief about yourself. We all have some area that we can work on improving!

How many of your thoughts are negative?

Do you see someone else's success and think "I can't do that", or start listing off the excuses of why they could do it, but you aren't able to?

Here are examples of what some of these poisonous thoughts may look like:

1. **The "Terrible Too's":** I'm too old, I'm too busy, I'm too out of shape, I'm too broke, I'm too dumb.
2. **The "Big But's":** I'd like to be healthy "BUT.. I don't have a gym membership", "BUT.. I can't afford a trainer", "BUT.. I like food too much", "BUT.. I'm married," "BUT.. I have kids," "BUT.. I travel a lot."
3. **The "I'm Not's":** "I'm not wealthy enough," "I'm not smart enough," "I'm not disciplined enough."

These thoughts all have to change if you want to be successful!

I'm not saying that there are no challenges on a fitness journey (or a journey to success in any other aspect of life)! There are!

Regardless of what the obstacle you're facing is, there is also a way around it, IF you want a new outcome.

The negative thoughts surrounding weight loss and healthy living in particular, don't hold up when you look at evidence.

There are healthy and fit people who have kids, who work full time, who travel a lot, who are well into their 50's, 60's and beyond, don't have gym memberships, don't have loads of money, don't have a personal trainer and who do love food.

NONE of these life circumstances prevent you from being a healthy person. When you come to that realization, it's a game changing revelation!

Action Step #2 - Check your attitude.

Personal attitude plays an ENORMOUS role in your ability to succeed. What is the frame you're using when you think of making healthy lifestyle changes?

When you think of losing weight or changing an exercise habit, do you see it as a sacrifice?

Do you feel like you would be "giving up" having "fun" in life if you changed your eating habits?

Do you tell yourself that you "hate" exercise?

Is your mindset one that believes you will be doing something that is not enjoyable?

These are all mental attitudes that will inhibit your progress and your long term success.

When we are rethinking fat loss, there are 3 areas that we need to make sure our thoughts and attitudes are pointed in a positive direction:

Mental Attitude towards FOOD:

Holding a negative perception of eating healthy foods will not likely lead to successful long term fat loss. This means saying and thinking that healthy food is "gross" or lacking in flavor or taste.

If you think something is gross, how long do you think you're going to adhere to eating it? Probably not for long!

It's true that people whose taste buds have been numbed by over consumption of a junk food, high salt, high sugar, high fat diet will have a bit of a shock to the palette when they switch over to consuming healthy whole foods!

But once the switch is made, the taste buds will change too. They can regain sensitivity and start to appreciate true taste and flavor. There is an entire world of delicious healthy foods that will not only make the body feel better, they will make it look better too!

Attitudes towards food CAN change!

The old thought process says that eating healthy is "gross". Stop that record from playing in your mind. Instead switch it to something like, "I love eating healthy foods that nourish my body and help me achieve my goals." Or it could be "I love finding new healthy foods to eat that I enjoy and that taste delicious."

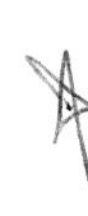

Come up with 5 positive attitude statements regarding the foods that you eat and start repeating them on a daily basis. Continue repeating those healthy statements to yourself as long as you need to until they are your "go to" thoughts. This is how you reprogram your mind.

Mental Attitude towards EXERCISE:

Maybe you are just fine making changes to food, but can't stand the idea of exercising.

Maybe you tell yourself that you "hate" exercise.

When you use the word "hate" you evoke an emotional response. The words we choose to use reflect what is happening within us.

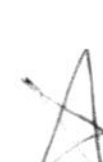

What is in the heart flows from the mouth. The word "hate" will elicit very strong negative emotions.

You can intentionally change up powerful negative words like this, to something less intense such as "it's not my favorite", or "I don't love it yet".

Just a simple switch in word use, will change how you feel about exercise, about eating healthy, about changing your lifestyle.

Take that a step further. You can really be intentional about changing your thought process by switching your words to the opposite of what you typically say.

If you think "I hate" something, change it to "I love". Just changing your self-talk will change how you feel and think about an activity.

This is a "fake it 'til you make it" approach. You may not initially feel what you're saying, but as you continue to say it, it will start to become a new reality for you.

If you say "I love exercise because it makes me feel strong and empowers me to enjoy the body that I live in," and "I love eating healthy because it makes my body feel good and allows me to change the way my body looks". These will have a powerful effect on your mind.

If exercise isn't your thing naturally, you can shift your perspective and look at it as a challenge that you're going to conquer, rather than something to dread. You may actually find that you enjoy it!

More often than not, I've heard people who once "hated" going to the gym, or doing cardio, discover that it has become their favorite part of the day.

Exercise in its many forms is excellent for physical health, strength of your bones, muscles, heart and lungs.

It's also fantastic for mental and emotional health, relieving stress, giving you the ability to clear your mind, gain focus and re-energize. It's a great tool for losing body fat (so long as nutrition is on track!), and also a great tool for maintaining fat loss for the long term.

There are many different modes of exercise too. There is a great variety of styles of workouts (I DO recommend that some form of strength training be a regular part of a healthy lifestyle for both men and women of all ages, literally for the rest of your life!), and many different methods of incorporating cardiovascular activity.

If you dislike one type of exercise, don't be afraid to experiment and try new things until you find something you enjoy.

I KNOW this intentional mental attitude shift works because

I've had to do it myself!

In 2005, when I changed my life around and determined to lose the 50 pounds that was dragging me down (mentally, emotionally and physically). I had to start waking up early to do cardio before my day began. I don't mind the cardio, but prior to that I would not have considered myself a "morning person."

Setting the alarm earlier and earlier so that I would have time to do cardio before my day began was a challenge. My preference would be to sleep in without an alarm, and take my time getting out of bed and going through my morning rituals. But if I wanted to get to my goal, that had to change.

I didn't want to get up early. But I wanted to achieve my goal. I knew that the action had to take place, and if I wanted to enjoy the action then I had to change my thoughts towards it.

I literally would go to bed and say "I can't wait to get up in the morning to do my cardio." I said it every night before nodding off to sleep. I repeated it in my mind over and over again. Anytime a grumble popped up, I chanted over and over to myself, "I love morning cardio."

Something strange happened.

I started to get excited about doing morning cardio. I anticipated getting to bed early so that I would be awake and ready to rock when the alarm went off.

Getting up in the morning took on a new meaning. It was now a chance to tackle a goal and make progress. I actually started to love that time in the morning. It became my favorite part of the day. I was able to move my body, get my thoughts together, work on problem solving for any issues that I was facing. I could tackle anything when I got up early and took the actions I needed to!

It was such a strange shift. Changing my thoughts, attitudes and words about something that I originally disliked, caused it to become one of my favorite things.

Our words direct our attitudes, attitudes impact our actions, and actions form the result of our life. They are so powerful!

Mental Attitude towards YOUR ABILITY TO SUCCEED:

This third area of attitude is a big one. As we discussed earlier, if you tell yourself that you are not capable of succeeding, that you "CAN'T" do something, then you will be right.

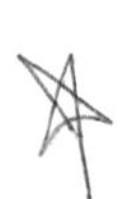

The truth of the matter is, you CAN make healthy changes to your life. NO. MATTER. WHAT. That's it. You have to start believing that for it to become reality.

Being healthy is a choice. I've never met a single person who told me their story, and I said…yes, you're right, you have no way to be a healthy person.

It's just never happened. There's ALWAYS a way.

There's a difference between saying you "CAN'T" do something, but in fact you simply don't WANT to, or aren't ready for the change.

If that's the case, then that is fine!

You should wait until you are READY to change, because that's when you will experience results that can last a lifetime. But OWN it. Don't say you "CAN'T" do it, because that's not true.

If it were a priority for you, then you would be more than capable.

For people who DO want it, and are ready for it. Change that "I can't" attitude as soon as you see it rearing its ugly head! Change it to "I CAN" and that's what is going to happen.

Keep in mind that "I CAN" doesn't mean perfection. It doesn't mean there aren't going to be challenges, obstacles, and potential setbacks. But that simple shift in mind set is going to power you through all of those things so that you achieve success.

Get your Mental Attitude in a positive place in all three of these areas and you will be on track to long term success for fat loss!

Action Step #3 - Shift the "sacrifice" mindset.

One of the negative thought patterns I've seen manifesting in many clients (and one that I had myself for many years), is the "sacrifice mindset." Shifting this mental pattern for myself is one of the biggest reasons that it's 14 years later and I have never gone back to my unhealthy eating habits.

Here's how this works.

You tell yourself that healthy eating and exercise is a "sacrifice".

You're "missing out" on eating this, that or the other thing if you make healthy choices. You won't have the same "fun" that others who are chewing and swallowing unhealthy junk foods are having. (The over-consumption of which would lead to living in a body that is unfit, sick, diseased in many cases, and that doesn't look or feel the way you want it to.)

When you do make a healthy eating choice, you have a martyr mentality, telling yourself that you made a big sacrifice by choosing health over something that would have tasted good for a few fleeting moments in your mouth.

If you tell yourself that making healthy eating choices is a sacrifice, and that you're "missing out" on filling your body with unhealthy food, then the chance of actually being a healthy person who gets to live in a healthy body, is slim to none.

This way of thinking, though extremely common, is narrow and limited.

Making a healthy eating choice is NOT a sacrifice. (It's actually a gift!) There is a FAR bigger sacrifice to consider.

The bigger sacrifice is when you decide that you don't want to "miss out" and choose to fill your body with junk.

When you choose unhealthy as a lifestyle (and I want to be clear that I'm not talking about treats and cheats in moderation as part of a healthy balanced life) here are some of the BIG things that you are sacrificing:

1. **Living in a body that you are comfortable in.**
2. **Living in a body that is free from the bondage to medication for diseases that are preventable and treatable through healthy lifestyle choices.**

3. **Living in a body that is high in energy.**
4. **Living in a body that you are confident to walk into a room of people with.**
5. **Living in a body that fits into the clothes that you want to wear.**
6. **Living in a body that enables you to enjoy intimacy with your spouse.**
7. **Living in a body that allows you to go on adventures and know that it will perform how you want it to.**
8. **Living with a mind that functions optimally and is more creative and problem solving.**
9. **Living in a body that allows you to keep up with the kids or grandkids.**
10. **Living in a body that feels good, serves you well, and isn't a distraction from your plans and purposes in life.**

These are BIG Sacrifices. These are far greater sacrifices than changing up what you're eating and moving your body on a regular basis.

Shift what you deem a sacrifice, and that will have a big impact on your goals and what you achieve.

This mind shift is SO important for the long term.

If you go on a "diet" and you tell yourself that you're sacrificing all the "good" foods during this time. You aren't likely to stay with this plan of action for long. You may do it for a while, but since you are telling yourself that you're making a big sacrifice, or that you're a martyr or a victim for making healthy choices, you WILL quickly go back to your starting point once you are finished.

I can't stress to you enough how important it is to take a look at where you are, and where you want to be, and then determine what the REAL sacrifice is.

It's not avoiding eating a cookie at the office, the bigger sacrifice is giving up your health to Type II diabetes. It's not skipping dessert at a restaurant, it's not being able to go out and play with your grandkids. (And let me be clear, I'm not saying that one cookie or an occasional dessert is the cause, I'm talking about making these choices on a consistent basis as a part of your normal eating patterns and lifestyle).

For me, I was sacrificing the big dreams and goals that were in my heart. I was sacrificing self-confidence and self-worth.

Years went by where I looked at where I wanted to be, and where I was, and didn't change, because I didn't want to "sacrifice" in regards to my eating habits.

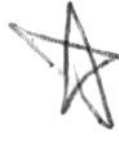

The moment I realized that not chewing and swallowing for a couple of seconds was not the sacrifice, that I was giving up so much more by filling my body with garbage, everything changed.

I'm not a martyr for choosing healthy. I don't do it because I "have" to. Because I don't' have to. I do it because I have the gift to make this choice, and I want to. I get to experience the big benefits and freedom that come as a result.

I recently received an email from someone who read my personal weight loss story. She told me that she had been advised to not "restrict" her eating choices because that would be mentally unhealthy. Yet ironically, she was trapped in an obese and sick body as a result of not having any discipline with her eating habits.

She is stuck in the sacrifice mindset that tells her developing discipline with her eating choices is the greater sacrifice.

This woman wanted to know how I did it. How did I "restrict" myself for so long.

I had to think about this for a moment. Because in my mind I don't see it as restricting myself. I see it as the opposite. To me, a restrictive life would be one where I didn't have a strong body that does what I want it to do. Living with restrictions would mean that I couldn't go for a hike whenever I wanted, or wear whatever I wanted, or be tied to a medication as a result of unhealthy choices.

I explained to her that I don't "have" to eat healthy. I "get" to eat healthy. It is a choice, and it's one that I make willingly and gladly. I make that choice because I don't want to be restricted from living out my dreams and goals by having a body that doesn't function or serve me well.

It's a freedom mindset.

Do you find yourself stuck in a negative sacrifice mindset?

Really evaluate it, make a list of the things that are on the other side waiting for you if you'll make change and commit. Then ask yourself what the bigger sacrifice is?

Action Step #4 – Protect your mind.

There is content and information that wants to be invited into your mind everywhere you look. Some of it good, some of it not so good, some of it down right bad.

Every television show, advertisement, post on social media, magazine or book, and even the people in your life, friends, family or co-workers, want to pour something into your mind.

Protecting your mind and having discernment over what is good and what is garbage is critical.

What you choose to allow into your mind will have an impact on the quality of your life.

You can spot a person who has filled their mind with negatives, with fears, with comparison, by what comes out of their mouth.

Pour in negative, out will come negative. Pour in positive, out will come positive. You have to decide what outcome you want from your life, and then choose to fill your mind up accordingly.

Here are some tips for protecting your mind:

1. **Pour in things that are empowering, motivating and make you want to go out and do something positive for yourself or others**.
2. **Practice gratitude**. One of the best ways to protect your mind is looking at your blessings and being grateful for them. A gratitude journal, where you take stock of the things in life you are thankful for, is a great way to get your mind to a positive and productive space.
3. **Reject messages or information that drags you down or pulls your mind to a negative place**.
4. **Careful of filling your mind with too much news, which tends to be negative in nature.** It's one thing to be informed of the affairs of the world, it's another to allow your mind to be immersed in negativity on a regular basis.
5. **Be discerning over which opinions of others you allow to have an influence on your life.** There are people who will lift you up, people who will give

constructive criticism that can help you grow stronger, and then there are critics who want to tear you down in order to make themselves feel better. The feedback from those who just want to tear you down, reject it and don't let it in.

6. **Be intentional with feeding your mind positive thoughts**. Write out 10 positive affirmations, in present tense (meaning don't say "I will" but say "I am") and read them aloud every single day so they become consistent thought patterns.
7. **Listen to the lyrics of your favorite songs and see what they are really saying**. One easy way our minds become flooded with negative messages is through music. Catchy lyrics repeat over and over, but make sure that they are not lyrics that set you up for negative thoughts.
8. **What you see, you can't un-see**. There are SO many choices available to watch on television or movies. Choose wisely!
9. **If you notice a negative thought floating through your mind, capture it and replace it with something new**. You may have to do this repeatedly as the new thought is established!
10. **Careful of social media**. This is listed as number 10, but is SO important. If you are NOT a confident person (yet). If you are not confident in your own life, your own skin, in who you are and your purpose in life, then be very careful with social media. Since social media portrays the "best" of people's lives, those who are currently insecure, will compare themselves and comparison is a killer. Comparison is a joy stealer and a contentment crusher. When you compare yourself to the social media lives of others, and what you are

seeing brings you down rather than inspires you or lifts you up, then UNFOLLOW or unsubscribe, or hide the content that brings you down. Take note of HOW you feel when you see the posts of others, if you find that they are discouraging, *then don't put them in your mind.*

Action Step #5 – Redefine Failure.

Success is NOT the absence of failure.

"Failure" is a part of the journey, so it is not something to be afraid of.

I've heard people say that they don't want to start a transformation journey, because they are afraid they will "fail.". Well, in all truth, YES, you're probably going to "fail" at one point or another!

It's not a matter of IF there will be moments of "failure", it's what you choose to do after those moments that will define your eventual success.

Failure isn't the end of the road. It's actually a growth and learning opportunity. It's a chance to evaluate what happened, determine if you produced the result you were hoping for, and if not, come up with a new strategy for next time!

The only way you truly fail is if you quit and don't keep trying. If you pick yourself back up, get things back on track, and just continue being persistent, then you haven't failed.

When it comes to a fat loss journey, the likelihood that every meal will be spot on, and you get every single workout in, or no old habits pop back up and suck you in for a moment, is unlikely.

Since it's probably going to happen, you can relax and just know that no matter what, you have the ability to get back on track.

People who are successful, are not that way because they never had challenges come up. They aren't successful because everything just fell perfectly into place and they breezed through.

On the contrary! Successful people are usually the ones who have failed miserably, have taken giant leaps of faith only to find their wings are not fastened securely and they come crashing to the ground.

In the world of finance, the greatest successes are typically those who have at one point been bankrupt or had a business failure.

In career, many who have achieved the highest levels of success in any industry have had multiple doors slammed in their faces, heard the word "No" repeatedly and been rejected on many occasions.

In the world of fitness, many of the top faces and leading names have experienced failure on different levels. Perhaps they were at one point failing in the area of physical health. Countless fitness experts (myself included!) have stories of at one point being overweight, unhealthy and unhappy in their lives.

What is it about failure that leads these people to even greater achievement?

If this is a common theme in the successful, how come every person who has failed in their life, isn't reaching these higher echelons of success?

They are successful because they failed, they dropped the ball, they got off track…and what did they do?

They got BACK UP. They didn't stay down. They didn't tell themselves that THEY were a failure. They did not claim that as their identity. Rather they saw that something didn't turn out as hoped, made mental notes and a plan of action for the future, and then just KEPT GOING.

If you have a failure, and you quit. You stay stuck. There's no chance of succeeding for the long term if you quit every time there is a set-back or perceived failure.

And guess what, you become STRONGER when you have failures. It's just like your muscles when you are training them. Train them until they fail and they will grow back stronger!

Don't be afraid to fail.

If you are afraid to fail, then guess what you need to do…FAIL. Because the way to overcome a fear of something is exposure.

When you fail and then get back up and keep going, you will start to see that it wasn't the end of the world after all, and that every day is a fresh start and a new beginning.

Failure is FEEDBACK. Redefine it and face it head on. Learn from it. Grow from it.

The day didn't go as planned and you didn't get a workout in?

Take a look at the next day and see where you can schedule it in and make it a priority.

Did you go on a trip and one cheat meal led to another and another and you ended up gaining weight?

All you have to do is get things back on track. There isn't a "last chance" to make a good choice for yourself until the day you're no longer on this earth!

Gave into temptation and ate something that set you back?

No need to be ashamed or embarrassed or to beat yourself up. Instead take a look at your goals, take a look at your thinking and why you decided to make that choice.

Do you need more powerful goals? Need to avoid places that will lead to temptation for a while until habits are stronger? Need to be more prepared with your choices so you aren't left feeling "stuck"?

Take that information and make a new choice next time.

The power of failure is all in the way that you view it, and where you choose to put your focus in the aftermath.

Those who look at themselves, something in their life, or the outcome of a certain event as a failure, and process that information as meaning that they are useless, not good enough, or not competent enough to pursue their goal, are the ones who are going to quit moving forward, curl up in a little ball of fear and stop making progress towards their goals.

These are the people who will remain status quo or less, they will stick with pathways that they feel are safe and have low risk of feeling that pain of failure again, these are people that will never attain a high level of success.

This does not have to be you!

There is a different way that failure can be viewed. A powerful and productive perspective that can get you so fired up, so determined, that you become unstoppable!

How do you define FAILURE?

Those who end up being ultimately successful at aspects in their lives are able to properly define levels of failure and assign an appropriate level of importance to them.

When you have, what you consider in your mind, failed at something, what are some of the emotions that you feel? What thoughts pop up?

Identifying these thoughts or emotions is one way that you can recognize the opportunity for growth and improvement. Here are a couple of the most common.

1. **Disappointment.** It's of course a natural human response to failure. But it is something you must be careful with. You can use disappointment in a negative way and decide that you should just not go after your goal any longer. OR you can change your perspective. Are there any positives that you took away from the situation? Did you learn anything from the situation that will allow you to improve or find an alternate route to the goal? Does the failure mean that a door is entirely closed or if you look around could there be a new window that has opened?
2. **Frustration.** This has the potential to be a great emotion if you properly direct it. When you feel frustrated, that means that you feel that you should have or could have achieved a goal. It bothers you that you didn't. This powerful emotion can lead you to going back to the drawing board, convinced that you CAN

achieve what you want, and develop a new strategy for getting where you ultimately want to be.

3. **Blame Game**. When you have "failed" at something, even if you may have every right to point the finger of blame on a person or situation, that isn't productive. EVEN IF, in your mind, it is completely the truth of the situation. And you may even be 100% right! But placing blame on anyone or anything else for failure is ultimately giving the power of the situation and the future of your success, to the person or event. To be the most successful, you don't want to give that power away. YOU want to have that power at all times, because ultimately it is YOU who are going to be the reason you are a success.
4. **FEAR**. This emotion is paralyzing. It is the one thing that will keep you grounded exactly where you are in life. It can prevent you from ever taking major strides towards goals and dreams that you wish you could attain. If you want something in life, you have to overcome your fear of failure and go for it. You need to SHIFT the fear. Rather than being afraid of doing something, think of what you will potentially miss out on if you don't go for it. Shift the fear so that you're more afraid of missing out on something amazing than you are of "failing" at the attempt. At the end of life, people rarely regret the things that they went after, they regret the things they were too afraid to go for.

Bring the failure on! Redefine it! Don't be afraid to look at the areas of weakness and be willing to do the work and make the changes to make them areas of strength.

To be the most powerful human being you can be, the most

successful, the most fulfilled, I encourage you to FAIL FEARLESSLY. Learn from every opportunity and use all of the knowledge and feedback you get to form yourself into the greatest success you can possibly be.

Chapter Review:

1. When you evaluate your self-talk, are your thoughts more negative or positive? Do you see areas that need improvement?
2. What are your current attitudes towards healthy eating, exercise and your ability to succeed? Are any adjustments needed?
3. How do you view healthy choices? Are they a sacrifice or something that you enjoy doing?
4. Are there areas where you need to protect your mind? What do you need to avoid or cut out in order to keep your mind in a healthy place?
5. How do you define failure? Is your definition empowering you to achieve your goals or holding you back from success? If it needs to change, how so?

Chapter 2.

INSPIRING GOALS:

And How to Set Them

Boring goals.

If you're bored by your goal, the likelihood of taking action to achieve it is slim to none. Why would you set a goal that bores you?

Sometimes it's because you feel like you are supposed to set it, maybe it's something that you feel societal pressure to achieve, but it's not an aspiration that truly comes from within you.

When it comes to creating a new healthy lifestyle, and achieving a goal as far as your physical body goes, a boring goal isn't going to do the trick. Your goals have to inspire you. The result has to be something that excites you to work for. The ultimate success that you desire has to have your attention.

Let me tell you why.

Success is all about consistency. That's true whether we are talking about your body, or a business, or a relationship, any area of life that you have goals you want to achieve.

And guess what, consistency can be (and IS in many ways) "boring". Say what? YES!! I said it!!! Consistency is often boring!!

If you've got a boring goal, and the path to getting there is going to be boring because it requires repetition, then boring plus boring will result in no action.

We've already discussed a lot about framing thoughts and words to more positive ones, so bear with me on this! Because I do believe that the belief that a process is boring can be shifted too!

The bottom line is this. Repeated positive habits, things that you do over and over and over again, lead to long term success. Once you've achieved success, you have to continue repeating the positive habits over and over and over again so that your success remains.

People who consistently achieve success from a physical health standpoint, understand that it isn't a one-time only event.

For example, I didn't lose 50 pounds and then think that the work was done. The 50 pound loss was the necessary first step, and it was an inspiring goal. But the day to day work to achieve it wasn't thrilling! It was monotonous for sure.

But what kept me going through the day by day little choices, that ended up in a big result, was having a goal so exciting to look forward to and experience.

Big, inspiring, motivating goals are worth the "boring". They are going to be worth the repetition, worth the consistency and worth the discipline.

The "boring" is what leads to the most exciting life.

Let's take a look at how to set blood pumping, heart pounding goals that are worth it to you!

Action Step #1– Identify where you are now and where you want to be.

You're planning a road trip.

When you go to Google Maps to find directions to a location, it needs to know where you ARE in order to tell you how to get where you'd like to be. Without this information, you won't have a clue what the route is and an approximation of how long it will take to get there.

This is the same with goal setting. If you don't have a clear picture of your current "address" then you won't be able to identify clear "directions" on how to get to your end goal!

Here's how to define your starting point and envision where you want to go:

1. **Buy a notebook or journal, or download an app that can serve as a journal on your phone (like Evernote or Samsung Notes).**
2. **Record your current situation**. Where are you physically, mentally, emotionally and spiritually? What is happening in your relationships, your work environment and your physical fitness activities. How is your confidence, your energy levels, your relationships? How is your health? Are you close to having to go on medication? Feeling run down? Lacking enthusiasm about life? This is a written "before" picture.
3. **If you have a physical goal, take actual "before" pictures**. Don't take headless photos of yourself, or fully clothed where you can't see your body. Before photos are information, they are where you are starting from!

Don't be afraid to be honest and real and just look the starting point right in the face. Regardless of your starting point, these are not about beating yourself up or feeling ashamed of past choices. They are just the marker for a brand new journey to a healthier version of you. They are a tracking point to look back on, so you can celebrate your progress and success and see how far you have come!

4. **Take measurements.** Since the path to success can be "boring" it is so important to have trackable ways of seeing your progress. There will be days where you lack motivation (even the most motivated people have these!). When you can look back and see where you started from, it will serve as fuel to keep you pushing forward.
5. **Figure out the destination!** Where do you want to be? Not just a number on the scale. Write out in detail what that new body feels like, what does that new life look like? What happens in every other aspect of your life in that place? How do you envision your relationships changing? How is your energy, your confidence? How is your day to day life going to be different? Take your time and be detailed! Take time to visualize it. Get a mental picture of what success will feel like. Even daydream about it!

You've got the mental picture of where you want to be. Now it's time to get clear on the specific goals that you are going to tackle.

Action Step #2 – Write out ACTION aspirations.

1. **Write out your aspirations**. Things you ASPIRE to. I think just changing what you call it changes how it feels. We use the word GOALS all the time, change it to ASPIRATIONS and that word feels so inspiring!
2. **Be specific**. Your aspirations need to be specific, so instead of saying that you are going to "lose weight" determine your starting point, and then determine a healthy goal to achieve in a time bound period. For example, I will lose 20 pounds of fat in the next 12 weeks, and I will do it by following my Hitch Fit plan and making healthy and consistent changes to my eating and exercise habits.
3. **Make sure that ACTION is required when you're writing out your goals**. To achieve it you have to DO something.
4. **Set a deadline**. Aspirations that are not time bound are typically procrastinated on. They stay in the "someday" pile instead of being bumped up to the "today and right now" pile. Even though a goal has a time frame to be achieved in, keep in mind that long term success isn't just one "event". It will still be ongoing consistency as you continue to develop new goals.
5. **Is it realistic?** Make sure that your goal is realistic for your starting point. 20 pounds of fat in 12 weeks is a healthy and doable goal. 50 pounds of fat loss in that time frame would not be a healthy goal for most people (unless starting weight is significantly high).
6. **REVIEW the goals every single day**. Whether they are on your phone. An app. A notebook next to your bed, or

even on your refrigerator. Regular review will help keep them TOP OF MIND.

7. **Record a wide variety of aspirations**. Narrow it down to the top one or two that you will be tackling first. Focus is so important for fulfillment of a goal, and having too many things that you are working towards simultaneously can dilute or delay progress in one focused area.
8. **Tell a friend**. Aspirations become real when you share them with others. Avoid sharing them with naysayers. Share them with people who will cheer you on and offer encouragement. That could be a good friend, a family member, a coach or a support group.

Action Step #3 – Define Your PATH.

You know where you are. You know where you want to be. But HOW do you get there? Here is where many people fall short.

New Years is a great example.

It's the beginning of a fresh year of life! Time to evaluate where you are at and where you want to be in a year from now. Weight loss is one of the most popular resolutions. Many people set themselves up for failure from the get-go by not taking action steps #1 and #2, finding out where they are and where they want to be.

Then there is the group that does take a look at the current situation, does know what the goal is. But they forget to get a map!

Instead they head out on the journey with no guidance or direction. They guess on which way to go, they have no idea what the best route is.

When you have no map, it's easy to get lost.

Getting lost is frustrating. Getting lost leads to quitting.

These are the people who buy the cheap gym membership, but then have no idea what equipment to use, or how to use it, or whether they should use weights or do cardio. And if they do weights and cardio, how much should they do, or how frequently should they do it?

These folks may jump on the bandwagon of the latest diet fad they've heard their friends talking about. Without knowing what they actually should eat, and how much and when to eat in order to get the result they are hoping for in their body.

The reason so many New Year weight loss resolutions fail, is because there is no defined path to get from point A to point B. If you want to arrive at your desired destination, get a map.

That being said, please know that ALL MAPS ARE NOT CREATED EQUAL!

Not every path will lead to your desired outcome. If you choose a map that is old and outdated, it may send you on a wild goose chase! If you take a path that takes you in a circle, you'll be back to square one.

Here are 3 tips for defining a path for your fitness goal, so you actually arrive where you want to be!

1. **Ask for directions!** Get help from someone who knows what they are doing. Careful here! There are a lot of people dispensing fitness myths and promises with no credible education on the topic, and no evidence to back up their

claims of success. Look for credible coaches, those who have a track record of integrity, and proven results. I'd of course be happy to help!

2. **The PATH for a Fitness Transformation should be Multi – Pronged**. It is NOT JUST ONE THING. It is not JUST a "diet" and changing eating habits. It is not JUST changing training habits and exercising more, but not making healthy eating changes too. If you want a true transformation. This is just like any other are of fitness. If you are very deconditioned and can't do ALL things right away, that is OK. You will start with what you can. Just understanding that you will need and want to do ALL things in order to achieve highest level of success. The path should include nutrition, exercise (both strength and cardio), and also address the importance of things such as hydration, sleep, and stress management.
3. **The PATH should be sustainable**. Beware of quick fix, short cut paths that promise fast results with minimal effort. These are the paths that will lead you around in a circle so you end up right back at the starting point! Red flags for paths to avoid are "diets" where you are eliminating food groups, or that have one certain food that is the "evil" food that everyone should avoid. Starvation is a red flag. Our bodies need fuel! If you look at the path and it's something you can't see yourself sticking to for the long term, then don't take it.

Action Step #4 – Create a reward.

Aspirations that have a reward system attached are much more fun to achieve! A reward is like a mile marker on your map. It breaks the journey down into smaller chunks, which helps keep you motivated.

Rewards come in a lot of forms. Some big and some small. Being able to put a check on your day and say that you made healthy eating choices and exercised gives a feeling of success, that is a reward!

Tracking calories burned and steps taken through fitness apps can be rewarding. If you're someone who likes a daily challenge, join some of the tracking apps that offer walking teams and get connected with others who are on their own journey. There are teams you can join and compete with one another (for example, seeing who takes the most steps in a certain time frame.) Working towards "winning" a challenge, or just beating your personal best is a form of a reward.

You can set mini goals and give yourself mini rewards along the way of your fitness journey. Maybe something special after each successful month of progress!

When you are on a fitness adventure and creating the healthiest version of you, avoid having food as a reward. Let me explain why.

Food is an amazing thing. One of the most amazing things about being a human being is our ability to choose our foods and enjoy them!

Food is fuel, but it is also for our pleasure. Not having it as a reward isn't because food is "bad". It's not. But having it as part of a reward system, if making healthy choices is something you have struggled with, can create a mental conflict. If food is the reward and your focus is on when you get to eat the foods that are "cheats", this can be a sign that your mind still is in a space of thinking that healthy eating is the sacrifice.

I encourage setting rewards that are not food so that the

journey isn't about living cheat meal to cheat meal. This keeps the mind stuck on food and takes focus off of the bigger benefits that are being reaped. It places emphasis on the thing that may have gotten you to an unhealthy place to begin with.

People who reward with food, often get stuck back in the same unhealthy habits as soon as they have achieved what they perceive as "the end." They reach the weight loss goal, reward themselves with food, and often get caught back up in the old habits and cycles.

A healthier choice, when you hit a milestone goal, (which may not be the ultimate end goal, but could be just the first big one) is to find a way to celebrate that solidifies the commitment to the new lifestyle.

Reaching the goal isn't "the end", it's actually just the beginning!

Here are some healthy, non-food, reward ideas.

1. **Take a trip or healthy active vacation.**
2. **Try a fun activity you haven't done before** (like rock climbing or surfing)
3. **Buy a new workout outfit or try on an outfit that didn't fit before, and now it does!**
4. **Go get a massage or spa treatment.**
5. **Try a new workout class that you have been interested in. (Either in person or this could be right at home).**
6. **Get a new piece of equipment for your home gym (doesn't have to be "new", just new to you!)**

One fun thing we do at Hitch Fit for our one on one clients who have gone through transformation, is set up a professional photo shoot where they get to be the fitness model! It is so much fun to see people who were once insecure and lacking confidence, get in front of the camera and show their stuff. It's an experience that makes them feel special and celebrated. It's an experience that they will not forget, and it's something that they will have memories (aka photos) to look back on and remember for years to come.

What are some rewards that you would look forward to?

Write out a list from both the small things, like a daily sense of wellbeing, to the big things, like a trip or photoshoot, that would make achieving your fitness milestones more fun and exciting!

We will dive a little deeper into the importance of rewards in chapter 5!

Chapter Review:

1. Where are you now and where do you want to be? (Remember to evaluate this from a physical, emotional, mental, spiritual and even relational standpoint.)
2. What are your ACTION Aspirations? Goals that excite you to achieve? How would achieving them change how you experience life?
3. How are you going to get there? What is your path?
4. What will your reward be (both for achieving small milestones and for the big ultimate goals!).

Chapter 3.

Fat Loss Focus:

End Scale Obsession

The scale.

For too many people it is the thing that determines if they have a good day or a bad day. It tells them if they are a success or a failure. It defines their self-worth.

Are you one of them?

Stop the madness! Stop giving that level of power in your life to something that doesn't deserve it. You are NOT the number on the scale. Do not let it define you.

That being said, it doesn't mean that the scale can't be a useful device for tracking progress and giving us information about our bodies. It can. When it's looked at for what it is, and used in a healthy, non-obsessive way.

As you embark on a transformation journey, shift your focus from the reading on the scale to fat loss. Make the goal a shift in your body composition, not just a "weight loss." Understanding the superiority of improving body composition, vs just losing a certain number on the scale, will help you develop healthier, more sustainable goals, with far less mental anxiety!

Action Step #1. Understanding Body Fat Percentage.

The number on the scale is a reflection of EVERYTHING that is part of your body. Your fat, muscle, tissue, organs, excrement, water, food that you just ate, etc. Scale weight does not discriminate. It just weighs everything that's on it. It doesn't give us any information as far as what your body actually looks like visually.

For example. Let's say we have two women who are both 5'7" and both weigh 140 pounds on the scale. One woman has a body fat of 16%, one has a body fat of 30%.

Do you think these two bodies look alike, even though they are the exact same height and weight? No. In fact they will look very different. The woman with 16% body fat will have much more tone on her body, and her actual body size will be smaller than the woman who is at 30%.

How can this be?

The reason for the difference in appearance is the fact that one woman has more lean muscle tissue. Muscle takes up less space in the body. A pound of muscle takes up a smaller amount of space than a pound of fat. Muscle is what gives the body shape. The woman with 30% body fat actually has 20 more pounds of fat on her body than the woman who is at 16%. Rather than focusing on achieving a number on the scale, a better goal is to achieve a healthier body fat percentage.

What is body fat percentage? This is the ratio of lean mass vs. fat mass on your body. It is different from BMI, which means Body Mass Index. BMI is simply a weight to height ratio, and tells us nothing about body composition. There are a wide variety of methods for measuring body fat percentage, and some more accurate than others.

Some of the most accurate, if you have access to them, are Bod Pod, DEXA Scan, Hydrostatic weighing, and Caliper testing by a skilled professional. Less accurate are body fat calculators online, hand held devices or scales. Even though the latter methods are less accurate, they can be valuable for tracking progress over time. They are typically more accessible and less expensive, and there is value in having a number that you can track progress with. [3]

Action Step #2 - Understand the Scale

You can overcome an obsession with the scale by understanding that the number is never stagnant. It will never be just one number at all times, and just stay that way for the rest of your life. It is going to go up and down, all day, every day, for your entire life.

Regardless of if you are a man or a woman, if you weigh yourself at 5 different times of the day, you are likely to get 5 different scale weights. Scale will go up after you eat or drink something. It will go down after using the restroom or after food has digested.

For women it will fluctuate during monthly menstrual cycles,

---

[3] The Hitch Fit Online Body Fat Calculator can give you an easy and trackable method of measurement: https://hitchfit.com/bodyfat-calculator/

the amount it varies can be on average 2-5 pounds depending on the woman. For some women this can happen during PMS, for some it is during the actual cycle. These scale fluctuations are from water retention, not from fat gains, and it's normal for them to occur every month (for as long as a woman is having regular cycles), no matter how lean you get!

Other things that cause scale shifts are hormone changes, lack of sleep, high levels of stress, constipation, hydration or dehydration, or eating something salty. If you ate something that doesn't agree with your digestive system which causes gas or bloating, that will also show up on the scale!

Any of these things will cause the scale to pop up or down. Since it isn't stable, it isn't reliable as the end all, be-all monitor of your progress.

It is fine to track the scale, but it should not be the determining factor of success. It also should not define you or put you in a bad mood for the day. If you have issues with the scale defining your day, then you may want to just stick with tracking inches and body fat losses.

This all being said, scale will move in a downward direction when you are losing body fat and changing your composition. If it is not changing at all, over a period of time, this could signal the need for an adjustment to your training and nutrition if there are also no reductions in body fat and inches.

Action Step #3 - Focus on Healthy FAT Losses not just "Weight" Loss.

When your sole focus is on losing scale weight fast, you are typically losing more than just body fat.

Popular diet fads will proclaim amazing and fast scale losses. They condition people to think that losing scale weight in a fast and furious way is a sign of success. But it's actually just the opposite.

When someone tells me they lost 20 pounds on a quick fix diet scheme, where they eliminated a food group, or starved themselves or did some type of "cleanse", my question is always "20 pounds of what?".

What did they actually lose?

Fast scale losses are not going to consist of just fat loss. Now, there can of course be some fat loss. But there is more to it than that.

One thing that people lose initially when they change their eating habits (and that can be as a result of either going on a fad diet OR if they are just changing over to healthier lifestyle habits) is water weight.

People who have poor eating habits are usually bloated on a daily basis without even realizing it. Changing eating habits will cause a reduction in water weight. This is why the first week of most new eating strategies or "diets" can lead to a larger than normal drop on the scale.

If the loss is a result of a starvation diet, then it's likely that a portion is lean muscle tissue.

If large losses continue on a weekly basis, the likelihood of continually losing lean muscle is very high. Someone who claims to have lost 20 pounds in a very short time most likely lost water weight, muscle weight and some fat weight.

Losing scale weight fast is actually EASY! All you have to do is starve yourself and do loads of cardio, and hallelujah, the scale will miraculously drop!

But the jubilation of fast losses can quickly turn to devastation when a couple weeks later the scale is back up even higher than it was before. Because the loss wasn't done in a sustainable or healthy way. There was so much focus on the scale, that body composition wasn't taken into consideration.

This is a big problem for yo-yo dieters.

They do the thing that leads to the big, gratifying in the short term, losses. But with those quick fixes comes muscle loss. The amount of muscle we have on our bodies impacts our resting metabolic rate. This is why losing muscle just to see the scale drop ends up backfiring in the long run.

When the quick fix or starvation method is no longer sustainable, even if the scale is lower, lean body mass is less.

Which means that when old eating habits return, metabolism is slower due to lower muscle mass, which makes fat gains even easier! When someone does this to their body over and over again, the body fat gets consistently higher and higher.

Losing body fat takes time.

When the focus is on fat loss rather than just scale losses, then big drops in a week are NOT a good sign. Fast losses are a signal that you're either not consuming enough or you're overtraining. Slow and steady is what wins the race for long term, sustainable fat loss.

What is healthy fat loss?

Generally speaking, if your goal is to lose weight and keep it off, you will want to aim for 1-2 pounds per week. It can vary slightly depending on the size of the person's body - for example someone who is small and has less fat to lose may lose less than a pound a week, someone who has a very large amount of weight may lose a slightly higher poundage in a week and it would still be healthy for them.

Body fat losses of about .5 – 1% per week are in a healthy range when you are in a transformation mode.

Patience is your friend when it comes to fat loss. Because a body transformation takes TIME. It won't happen overnight.

Often I hear clients express that weight gains crept up on them over the course of several years, sometimes it's been decades or a lifetime. It didn't come on overnight, it's not going to come off overnight.

The key to a fat loss that is permanent, is taking things slowly.

A fat loss journey is typically NOT a straight line, it is more of a zig zag. This is because there are many other factors that come into play (for example, stress, sleep, hormone shifts). That means some weeks may be a little more, and some weeks may be a little less! That also means there may be weeks where you don't see a loss at all. BUT there may be changes in your inches or a slight drop in your body fat.

If you give up or quit because you have a week where the scale didn't do what you wanted it to, or didn't move as much as you wanted it to, then you aren't likely to get to your goals for the long term. Be patient with your body. Being impatient can actually increase stress and anxiety, and that can work against your fat loss goals.

To feel successful, set smaller, short term, doable goals. Celebrate these mini successes and watch them add up to a big success in time!

Action Step #4 – Understand Importance of INTENSITY.

Cardio Intensity. It's the secret ingredient to losing more body fat, but did you know it can also be a key to living a longer life?

It's true!

Let's talk about the losses in body fat first.

Have you ever been to a gym and seen people doing cardio, but they aren't breaking a sweat, aren't breathing hard, and can easily carry on conversations with others around them, or read, play on their phone, or be engrossed in a television show? How much of an effect do you think this cardio is having for the individuals fat loss goals?

Probably not much.

There was a myth that was popular for years that claimed that people would only burn fat if they did low intensity cardio. It's not true. It's been debunked in study after study. Yet I still hear people use it as a reason to not kick the cardio up a notch and really push themselves to get the heart rate elevated. The myth came from the discovery that more fat was mobilized at lower cardio intensity.

What does that mean? Picture a fat cell. A cell that is filled with triglycerides. Those triglycerides can be used for energy if they can be "mobilized" or broken down, or for simplicity, released from the fat cell.

The release or break down process is called lipolysis (a result of the enzyme lipase) and one of the ways that lipolysis occurs is when the body needs energy, such as when you're doing cardiovasacular activity or other exercise. The triglycerides are then used for energy. (The fat cell itself does not excrete from the body, it stays there, and can be refilled with fat).

When doing lower intensity cardiovascular training, studies showed that more triglycerides were mobilized, and a higher percentage of the calories burned during the low intensity exercise were burned from fat. Makes sense then. We should do low intensity cardio, right?

Not so fast.

When you do a higher intensity level of cardio, you burn MORE calories overall in a shorter time frame. Even if a lower percentage of the calories burned are fat calories, you still burn MORE fat overall simply because you utilized more energy.

Here's another fun fact.

Did you know that you BREATHE fat out? It's true. Those triglycerides, once they have been used for energy, have to be released from the body in the form of waste products such as sweat, saliva, urine, feces, and your breath. A study done by Ruben Meerman and Andrew Brown[4] discovered that MOST of the work to excrete the fat was done by the lungs, through exhalation. Yes, you literally are breathing out your fat!

When you exercise at higher intensity levels, you utilize more oxygen, you exhale more carbon dioxide. You take more and faster breaths in and out. That means you are literally excreting more fat when you breathe heavier and harder. Now, that doesn't mean to hyperventilate! But, it does mean, that if you have fat loss goals, you're going to reach them more efficiently and effectively by kicking the intensity levels of your training up a notch.

What about longevity?

Studies show that there is a direct correlation between higher VO2 Max capability (that means the maximum amount of oxygen that an individual can utilize during exercise) and mortality. The higher VO2 Max, the higher your aerobic capability and endurance. It's an indicator of a high level of cardiovascular fitness AND a chance at leading a longer life.

The less fit you are, the more opportunity you have to improve your VO2 Max.

Another mortality indicator is Heart Rate Recovery (HRR). This is basically the speed at which your heart rate recovers to a normal pace after it has been elevated. The faster that your heart is able to recover, the better. A speedy HRR is an indicator of cardiovascular health and a longer life span.

Want one more?

[4] "When Someone Loses Weight, Where Does the Fat Go?
(BMJ 2014;349:g7257) – Meerman & Brown

Let's take a look at resting heart rate. This is the beats per minute that your heart performs at rest. When your heart is healthy and strong, your beats per minute are lower, because a healthy heart doesn't have to work as hard as an unhealthy heart.

The way to see improvement in all three of these longevity indicators is, you guessed it, exercise. Specifically, intense exercise that makes your heart work harder, and as a result become even stronger! Keep that in mind in your next workout, see if you can kick things up a notch! Progress yourself little by little, not all in one day, improving your training capability will take time and consistency too! Those extra efforts are going to add up!

**If you have a medical heart condition or health issues that would contradict high intensity exercise, see your physician for guidelines on what intensity levels are appropriate for you.*

Chapter Review:

1. Do you understand body fat composition vs. the number on the scale?

2. Does the scale control how you feel about yourself? If yes, what are some strategies you can use to change the emotional attachment to that number?
3. Now that you understand fat loss vs. scale loss, what do you think a good fat loss goal would be? What methods of measurement do you have available to track it?
4. How would you rate the intensity of your workouts (so long as you don't have health contraindications to intense exercise). Do you feel that you are doing your best or do you see areas where you can improve?

Chapter 4.

Food Anxiety:

And How to Overcome It

You can't turn on the television, read a magazine, look at your phone or talk with friends without hearing about the latest fads, elimination diets, or "bad" foods.

It goes something like this:

This food causes inflammation...you can eat this...no you can't... you should eat that...no you shouldn't.

You should eat meat. You shouldn't eat meat. You shouldn't eat carbs, you should only eat carbs. You should eat only fats, you shouldn't eat much fat.

All of the chatter (and a lot of it misinformation), is causing people to have high anxiety over what they are eating.

They are confused about what to eat and what not to eat, and some people have so much stress over what to eat that they are actually gaining weight!

Another issue causing anxiety is believing in a "bad food", and then eating it, and then feeling that you need to punish yourself for the poor choice, or "make-up" for it. Or perhaps you tell yourself that you "failed" your diet, so you may as well give up!

This seems like some serious mental stress to me!

Cortisol levels can increase with stress and this can fight against fat losses. Those who are prone to emotional eating, may be triggered to eat even more when they experience food anxiety.

How do we stop it?

Action Step #1 – Stop Stressing.

This is probably easier said than done if you are someone who has had anxiety over food for a long time. But seriously, for your best health, physically and mentally, stop stressing!

First, you can stop stressing about their being just ONE way to achieve fitness goals. There isn't!

There are fit and healthy people who eat MANY different styles.

Be careful of following fitness evangelists who tell you that there is only one way to eat to get a fit and healthy body. It's just not true. Think of a vegan vs. someone who eats a high fat diet. Both may obtain fat loss, and both may claim that they feel great with their preferred style of eating. These are two OPPOSITE eating strategies, and both can lead to a desired result, IF they can be sustained in a healthy way for the long term.

Relax and know that there isn't just one way, there isn't a one size fits all style of eating that everyone needs to do. There isn't one evil food group that you have to avoid forever to be healthy.

Next, stop stressing if you get off track.

Let's say you've committed to a healthier lifestyle, but you eat something that doesn't support your goals. You do NOT have to punish yourself for it, you do NOT have to try to make up for it. But as discussed in the section on "failure", you can use it for feedback and learn from it.

Once you've made a choice, you won't be able to go back in time to change it. It's done. Move on. It's ok to move on. BUT take time to reflect.

In all my years as a coach, I would say that less than 1% of clients have a journey that is "perfect."

I work with online clients all over the world, and have been at it for over a decade. I will leave it to you, to imagine how many messages I've received over the years from someone who was on a good track, making great choices, and then "something" came up. An event, a trip or celebration, or something tragic like a death, illness or loss of some type. Life threw a curveball, and they made a choice they didn't feel great about.

What is my response?

Typically, it's "don't stress." But also, don't miss out on this learning opportunity.

If things fall off track, all you have to do is get right back on. If your good habits fell to the wayside for a week or months or even years, and you decide you want to re-commit to them, then guess what, you can.

It's never too late. One choice that's in conflict with your goals doesn't define you.

Here are some questions you can ask yourself so you can stop stressing and get back to making progress towards your goals.

1. **Why did I make this choice?** Was it because of temptation or peer pressure or lack of preparation?
2. **Where did the choice lead?** Did it get me closer to where I want to be or did it push me further away?
3. **How did it make me feel physically?** Did my body feel well or did it feel ill?
4. **What are some strategies or preparations I could do next time in order to stay on track towards my ultimate goals?**

Instead of stressing, you can use this opportunity as a way to learn more about yourself, and come up with strategies that will empower you for the future. Then anticipate that challenge coming again, but now it is a chance to practice and implement your new strategies. It becomes something fun to look forward to!

Action Step #2 - Think Long

Before you embark on any new plan for fitness, think about the long term.

If you think that cutting out all your carbs is a good idea, are you going to do it for the rest of your life? If you're thinking about just eating fats, will you do it for the rest of your life? If you're thinking of cutting out gluten (and you don't actually have Celiac disease or a gluten allergy), are you going to do it for the rest of your life? If you're going to rely on a food service to deliver all your meals, are you going to do it for the rest of your life?

If the answer is yes, then go for it. But if the answer is no, then find a new strategy. Because if it's not something you can do for the long term, you have to ask this question.

THEN WHAT??

If you enjoy eating carbs, and aren't going to cut them out for the rest of your life, but go on a carb elimination diet to lose weight fast....then what?

What I've seen often as a result of this approach is that a person gets to the point where they can't stand not having carbs anymore and they go the opposite direction and over indulge (regain weight quickly), and then beat themselves up mentally for not being able to stay on track. This isn't healthy for your body OR for your mind.

Let's say you decide to rely on a food service to send you meals. You don't learn about the foods you're putting in your body, or know how to go to a grocery store and choose good food options. You don't take the time to understand how to read nutrition labels, or learn what portion sizes are and how to choose ones that are right for you. You don't learn how to prepare your own foods so that you have control over what you're putting in your body. When you no longer can afford to have the food service or it's not available or you're tired of it...then what?

Well, you're back to square one. Back to not knowing what to eat, when to eat it or how much of it to eat. Back to not knowing how to choose your own foods and give your body what it needs in order to achieve your goals.

If new eating habits weren't developed, and you weren't intentional about going through the education process as far as learning about the foods that you're putting in your body, then it's too easy to fall right back into the old patterns.

When you're thinking long, think about what you will stick with. How can you see yourself eating for a lifetime?

LEARN the skills that you'll need, in order to be independent with your eating choices. Pre-made meals and food services can be GREAT if you're a busy person who needs help staying on track. BUT, make sure before you resort to these, take the time to learn about your foods.

With a bit of intention, and good direction, it doesn't take long to learn about the foods that will keep your body looking and feeling great. That way you have the knowledge in your mind that you need for life. You aren't relying on anyone else for your success.

Relax, and find an approach that works for YOU.

Action Step #3 – Avoid (Unnecessary) Elimination

I know that elimination diets are all the rage.

Eliminate carbs. Eliminate gluten. Eliminate soy. Eliminate dairy. Eliminate meat.

Seems like everywhere you look there is a new report or best-selling book that has the secret to weight loss, and it's eliminating some "evil" food from your diet. They add some snippets from a research study in there (often cherry picked data that often doesn't even give the full results or scope of the study!) to make it seem like they've discovered the ultimate answer!!

What we've got out there now are all these eating theories, some of which are in total contradiction to one another, all touting that they are the magic eating style that will work for everyone.

Truth is, there are studies to support both sides of the coin for most foods.

There are people who are healthy fit and lean who eat gluten, there are healthy, fit and lean people who don't eat gluten. There are healthy and fit people who eat dairy, there are fit and healthy people who don't eat dairy. There are fit and healthy people who eat meat, there are fit and healthy people who don't eat meat.

The chaos and confusion over people thinking that they need to eliminate certain foods to be "healthy" is giving people food anxiety! People with no need to eliminate a food from their diet are doing it because of hype that they've heard. This makes things harder than they need to be.

My advice is to avoid unnecessary eliminations from your diet.

That being said, some people NEED to eliminate certain foods or even food groups due to disease or allergies or medical conditions. People who have Celiac disease for example, need to eliminate gluten completely from their eating strategy. Not just for the short term, but for the long term.

If people have an actual gluten allergy or sensitivity, they would want to cut back or eliminate it as well. If someone suspects that they have a gluten allergy, don't self-diagnose! Go and get it checked. Self-diagnosis when it comes to this allergy can be dangerous. If you suspect you have an issue with gluten, you need to go and see if you have Celiac disease or not. If you self-diagnose, and cut it out for a while, and then get lax and add it back in here and there, even small amounts can cause a lot of damage. Also, if you cut out gluten prior to having a test for an allergy done, it can impact the test results! If you suspect it. Check it.

People who do not have an actual gluten allergy or sensitivity, do not need to eliminate it from their diets.

New studies are showing that people who do not have gluten related disorders, but have eliminated gluten from their diets, are experiencing nutritional deficiencies in calcium, fiber and B vitamins.[5] [6]This doesn't mean that eating high amounts of gluten is a good idea either! When you're eating a balanced nutrition style with healthy whole foods, a majority of those foods won't contain gluten to begin with.

It's important to understand that just because something is "gluten free" or "vegan" that doesn't mean that it is a healthy choice. These foods can be highly processed, be loaded with sugar or high in unhealthy types of fat!

If you have a sensitivity to dairy or lactose intolerance, then by all means eliminate dairy. Or if you simply don't like dairy, then it's fine to eliminate it.

If you don't have sensitivity or allergic response to dairy, then you don't need to eliminate it. Again, that doesn't mean eating

---

[5] Golley S, Baird D, Hendrie GA, Mohr P. Thinking about going wheat-free? Evidence of nutritional inadequacies in the dietary practices of wheat avoiders. Nutr Diet. 2019 Jul;76(3):305-312. doi: 10.1111/1747-0080.12521. Epub 2019 Mar 14. PubMed PMID: 30873744.

[6] Diez-Sampedro A, Olenick M, Maltseva T, Flowers M. A Gluten-Free Diet, Not an Appropriate Choice without a Medical Diagnosis. J Nutr Metab. 2019 Jul 1;2019:2438934. doi: 10.1155/2019/2438934. eCollection 2019. Review. PubMed PMID: 31354988; PubMed Central PMCID: PMC6636598.

loads of dairy! But it also means you don't need to unnecessarily eliminate a food that does have a lot of benefits, including being high in quality protein, if it's something that you enjoy.

Lean meats such as chicken, turkey and fish are excellent sources of protein, valuable for building, maintaining and repairing lean muscle tissue, and helping with feelings of satiety. However, if you don't want to eat meat because of ethical or moral reasons, or because you simply don't like it. No problem. You can achieve fat loss success with a vegetarian or vegan style of eating too.

Don't make things harder on yourself by eliminating foods unnecessarily that are perfectly fine to include as part of a balanced long term nutrition strategy.

Over the years, I've seen that a balanced approach to eating with flexibility and variety of foods leads to the highest chance for sustainability for the long term.

Action Step #4 - Watch Your Language

Eliminate anxiety about your food choices by watching your language.

When you say you "can't" have something, then you automatically set yourself up to crave and want it.

In a social setting, if you tell people that you "can't" have something because you are on a "diet", more often than not, the people around you will do everything they can to encourage you to eat it (which leads to even more mental stress!).

It may not be a conscious attempt at sabotaging you, but when people feel insecure with themselves or want to justify their own choices, they will typically try to get you to make the same ones that they are.

Change the talk and SPEAK TRUTH.

The truth is that you CAN eat anything that you want. No one is forcing you to make a healthy choice. You are fully capable of eating anything and everything that you desire. You CAN eat pizza and ice cream and drink beer all day, and that is totally your choice.

However, every choice leads to a result or consequence. So if you have a goal that is important to you, it's not about "can't" have something, it's about "don't want" something because it doesn't align with what you say that your goal is for yourself.

In social settings, rather than saying you "can't" eat something, just say that you don't want it, or that you "don't like" it. Rather than saying you're trying to "lose weight", say that you're making healthier choices for yourself because you feel better when you do!

This simple change in language will be truthful, will help you avoid the mental pressure that comes when you tell yourself you "can't" have or do something, AND people will be far less likely to pressure you to try and eat it.

Ultimately, your choices are your own. Regardless of what anyone else says to you, you still have to own that decision. Your choices only impact your body, no-one else's. Don't use peer pressure as an excuse to make choices that push you further from your goals. BUT, learning some ways to avoid unneeded temptation will certainly help you maintain your resolve.

Chapter Review:

1. Are you stressed about your food choices? Confused about eating "bad" foods? What are some new thought patterns towards food that you could work on developing to stop stressing?
2. If you're thinking long about your eating and exercise habits, can you continue with them (at least the majority of the time)? If not, what part of what you're doing is not sustainable? What do you think would be sustainable for you?
3. Have you unnecessarily eliminated any food groups? Are there healthy food options that you'd like to add back into your nutrition that would give you more variety and flexibility of choice?
4. What type of language do you use in regards to your eating habits? Can you change it to empowering words? How can you change the language you use in social settings to avoid peer pressure from saboteurs?

Chapter 5.

Power of Habit:

And How To Create Good Ones

Over the years I've seen people start making healthy choices, then revert back to old ones. They go on a diet, then go off the diet, reversing any progress that was made. They begin a plan, take a few steps forward, then quit and abandon their goals. I've seen people say they want change, and then never even take the first step!

One of the common excuses I hear from people who don't start, who quit or revert right back to old habits is that they "Don't have the willpower".

But is willpower really the key to success?

It's not!

If you rely on willpower alone, then the chances of permanent, long-term success are slim. We are human, and we ALL have good days and bad days, we all have challenges that come up, we all have emotions and feelings. Things that can distract us from our "will" or reduce our "will".

The key to long term success is HABITS.

When something is a habit, you do it on autopilot. You do it because it is a part of who you are and what you do. You do it regardless of what your level of "will" is, because it is routine.

Studies done by neuroscientist Wolfram Schultz[7] were revolutionary in understanding habit development. He discovered that the first step in habit development is having a cue, which leads to a routine, which generates a reward.

Action Step #1 – Create Healthy Cues, Habits and Rewards.

If you are going to start exercising in the morning, have your workout clothes and music ready. When you wake up in the morning and see them sitting there, that's your cue to put them on and get your workout done.

A cue for new eating habits could be to set alarms for yourself throughout the day, so you remember to eat your meals. Soon your body and mind will understand this cue. When the alarm sounds, it's time to eat!

The cue will be the set up for your new habit or routine.

The response to a cue is the same for both good and bad habits.

A cue for a smoker could be seeing a pack of cigarettes, or the clock hitting a certain time of the day that they normally go out for a smoke. For someone who regularly consumes fast food, seeing a sign for their favorite fast food joint, or smelling one of the foods from that place, can be a cue. The cue occurs, and then they go through the routine, and then they reap a reward.

We discussed rewards in an earlier chapter, they are important to have as motivators for achieving a goal, but now we are going to take a closer look at how they come into play when we are developing healthy habits.

---

[7] "The Power of Habit: Why We Do What We Do What We Do in Life and Business" by Charles Duhigg 2014

The reward can be any number of things.

At the fast food joint, it would be the few seconds of chewing and swallowing. This is something the brain says gives pleasure. (Even if the longer term outcome is actually negative, such as disease, sickness, guilt and not feeling well in the body you live in).

One of the biggest rewards for our brains is the fulfillment of a craving. The strong desire to fulfill cravings is one of the main reasons people engage in harmful behaviors that are destroying their health and literally killing their bodies.

When you stop a bad habit, it's best to replace it with a good habit. That way you won't have a void. For example, if you usually go out for a smoke break, rather than having nothing to do, find a friend who will go out for a walk with you during that time instead.

As you begin creating new cues and habits, what are some healthy rewards that are appealing to you? For people who experience long term, permanent fat loss, here are some of the non-material rewards that they begin to crave:

1. **Experiencing life differently**. Living in a body that feels strong, healthy and fit is an amazing feeling. Being able to go for a hike when you want to, take on a physical challenge and KNOW that your body is going to be able to perform is incredibly rewarding.
2. **Endorphin release**. Exercise produces the secretion of the endorphin hormone which boosts mood and general feelings of well-being. Endorphins are boosted after a variety of activities, including challenging physical exercise like strength training or cardio.

3. **Sense of accomplishment**. It feels good to check things off your daily "to do" list. When you've committed to healthy living habits, and can, at the end of the day, check off the commitment to make healthy eating choices and exercise, that creates a feeling of satisfaction and fulfillment. When you have made the commitment and then don't follow through, that can lead to the opposite feelings of disappointment and frustration or guilt.
4. **Shopping and enjoying it**. This one is especially true for women, but it's a big deal for men too! To walk into a store, try on clothes that you like, and have them fit you well is an amazing feeling.
5. **Only trying on ONE outfit in the morning**. I work with a lot of business women, so I know this one is true! It is a great reward to go in your closet in the morning, find an outfit that you like, and know that you are going to like how you look and feel when you wear it that day.
6. **Excitement to track progress**. When you are tracking your physical stats including body fat, inches and scale weight, an excellent reward is when you see positive progress in those stats after you have made good choices to achieve them!
7. **Energy.** This is one of the best rewards of caring for your body. When you get home after a long day of work, and still have energy to spend time with your children or your spouse, rather than being so tired you have nothing left for them, that is one of the most fulfilling rewards you can ask for!
8. **Confidence walking into the room.** When you walk into a room full of people, and you feel good about yourself, feel strong, healthy and comfortable with how your body looks, you will enter with your head held high.

9. **Picture satisfaction.** To be in photos, whether it is family pictures, or memories being made with friends, and feel like you're excited to see the images is an empowering feeling. You no longer feel the need to hide in the back or behind anyone or anything.
10. **Look great naked.** When you feel like you look great naked, and have no problem letting your spouse see you in your full glory, in full light, that is a game changer for intimacy levels in your relationship!

As you engage in healthy habits, you'll start to expect the reward that's coming. The game changer is when the expectation becomes an actual craving for the reward. That's when a good habit becomes a permanent part of your life. You crave the good feelings, you crave the accomplishment, the confidence or energy or health, and that makes you WANT to engage in the behavior over and over again, for the rest of your life.

As you can see, being successful for the long term is not JUST willpower. It's habit.

Don't get me wrong. Willpower is great AND important.

It's just like a muscle. When you determine to make a good choice, even in the face of temptation, you will also gain strength of willpower. This is beneficial and extremely helpful for goal achievement!

But, if you want to transform your body, and keep your progress for the long term, then stop thinking that the greatest key is developing super human willpower (because few people get to that level, but many can be successful!).

Get to work today on setting cues, taking action and following the routine (whether that is making a healthy eating choice or exercising). Take stock of the rewards. Get excited about those rewards, focus on those rewards, and when you get to a point where you are craving them, you will have healthy habits set on autopilot for life.

Action Step #2 - Practice, Practice, Practice.

As you're developing new habits, you initially have to pay attention and be intentional. You have to PRACTICE them. You have to practice the habit even when you don't feel like doing it. You have to practice consistently, just like you would if you were learning to play a new instrument. You practice until you are good...and then great at the performance!

Think of when you start a new job. Initially you may not know what to do, where things are, or what the daily flow is. But as you learn the day to day procedures at your work environment, you eventually do them on auto pilot without even thinking. It takes far less mental energy once those habits are developed.

That's the point you want to get to with healthy habits. When you have practiced them consistently, then no matter what life throws at you, you STILL make the healthy choices because it is your habit. That doesn't mean things are perfect, but it means that the habit is so engrained in you, that you find a way to make it work (at least to the level of degree that you're able to depending on the circumstances), no matter what happens to try to throw you off course.

Remember that "bad" habits have the same flow as far as cue, routine and reward. Do not let those old ones come creeping back in!

Back to willpower for a moment.

Since willpower will strengthen with use, don't be afraid of going into situations where you will HAVE to put it into practice. You may not do this at the very beginning of a transformation journey, but as new habits begin to develop, don't be afraid to try them out in settings that will be a norm for the rest of your life.

For example. Go to a social event where you know there will be foods that were once stumbling blocks for you.

Let's say it's a table of cookies and sweet treats. In the past you would have bee-lined it straight to the table to load up. Or maybe your go-to old habit was a bit more subtle, you saw the table and then thoughts were filled with how to get over there to eat something without people noticing. Maybe you casually struck up a conversation with someone near it, grabbed a treat here, and then another treat there.

Regardless of what the old habit was, strengthening willpower, and creating and practicing a new habit for these situations is going to be critical for long term success.

The more you put good choices into PRACTICE, the easier they will become.

I believe social situations, vacations, celebrations and things that are unexpected are actually GOOD when in a time of transformation. Since you're giving so much more intentional thought to your goals, and the choices that get you to them, it is an excellent chance to practice making great choices, while you're strengthening willpower and creating strong habits.

The new habit in this case may be making the choice IN ADVANCE that you are not going to eat any of the cakes or cookies, and then following through on that choice. You will leave the party without having eaten anything that doesn't align with your goals.

Make note that the mindset was not that you CAN'T eat anything at the table. Because that would be a lie. You of course have the choice to eat whatever you want to. It is also your choice to practice your new habit, and leave with a feeling of achievement and a little more willpower strength than you walked in with!

Action Step #3 - Habit Continuation – "Sustainability".

Once you've developed habits, you must CONTINUE them for the long term.

This is why, prior to beginning any fat loss journey, you evaluate its sustainability, and if you believe you will stick to it for the long haul, at least the majority of the time.

What is sustainable for you?

You must ask this question because the only way to achieve your goals and then SUSTAIN them for the long term is going to be by continued habits.

If you go back to the old habits or "bad" habits, then your body will go back to its former condition. If you dropped body fat by making healthier eating choices and exercising regularly, and then you STOP eating healthy, or stop strength training regularly, then you will LOSE your progress. You will be back at square one.

Strength training is something you will need to do, literally for the rest of your life. That doesn't mean you have to do it every day or for long hours, but it will need to be a part of your routine in one form or another.

You will not be able to strength train for just a few weeks or a few months, and then stop, and expect to maintain high levels of strength and lean muscle.

I have a lot of women come to me and say they want to be "toned". All that they are saying is that they want to have lower body fat, and to be able to see the shape of the muscle that is underneath the skin and fat. The strength training is what develops that muscle that is under the skin. If they stop strength training, after doing it for a while, the body just goes back to being soft and squishy.

I had a client who reverted back to old eating habits after going through transformation, and sure enough, her body fat went back up to a place where she wasn't comfortable.

Essentially, she just went back to eating whatever, whenever. She went back to no discipline with her habits.

She told me that she needed something that she could "sustain."

But it made me think, what does sustainability really mean to her?

Think of this. You want your body to look and feel a certain way, but you're not willing to have discipline with your eating habits. You tell yourself that what is "sustainable" behavior for you is being able to eat whatever and whenever. If that is the behavior you can sustain, then the condition that will sustain in your body will be a higher body fat. The sustainable condition will not be a body that is lean and fit.

You can't have sustainability without self-discipline. It has to be understood that a level of self-discipline (which is a GOOD thing), will be required for you to keep yourself in a place where you are comfortable. If you're looking for sustainability without self-discipline, it doesn't exist!

I can certainly understand the lack of sustainability if the route to fat loss consisted of a lot of fancy recipes, cooking times or eliminating complete food groups. That would be hard to stick with for people who are on the go, with busy schedules.

If you took a balanced, slower approach to fat loss, kept in good variety and flexibility with your food choices, found foods that you enjoyed, learned how to make healthy choices even when eating out, and learned really quick, fast and easy options for foods to eat throughout the day, then sustainability IS an option IF you're willing to stay disciplined, at least the majority of the time.

Please know that when you lose weight, your body will initially want to return to its starting point. To stay in a place where you feel great, you are going to have to fight back. The way you wage that battle is through consistency with the habits you've learned, and self-discipline.

That being said, the level of adherence, when you're focused on maintaining progress, is lower than when you are in a transformation mode. This is good news! This means that when the goal is sustaining, you have more flexibility, since you're trying to keep your body in the same place.

During transformation, at Hitch Fit, we encourage people to be at a 90% or higher adherence level for the most efficient progress. In other words, be an "A" student. That doesn't mean that being a "B" student doesn't result in transformation happening, it still can and does, it just takes a little longer is all!

When your body is in a good place that you are comfortable and confident, then to maintain or sustain typically requires being at about 80% adherence or being a "B" student. If you slip down into the "C's", that's when you start going back to your starting point.

Tips for Sustainability:

1. **Evaluate a plan of action in advance to see if it something that you will be able to stick to**. If it requires hours of food preparation, or fancy recipes, or eliminates a food group entirely, will you be able to stick with it?
2. **Lose body fat slowly and steadily and avoid fast losses**. The longer a transformation takes, the more engrained the habits can become, and the more of a lifestyle it will be.
3. **Shift gradually from a transformation style of eating to a maintenance/sustainability style of eating**.
4. **Stick with the habits that you have learned at least 80% of the time**. If time is an issue for you, stick with quick, healthy and easy options that will keep you on track.
5. **Learn and practice making healthy eating choices at restaurants and when in social situations.**
6. **Keep an eye on things!** If the scale and body fat start creeping back up, don't wait until it is a 20 pound regain, reign things back in by tightening up the nutrition (cutting back on treats and cheats which have become too frequent is usually the culprit).

7. **Drop training volume down to a maintenance level.** In general will be weights anywhere from 2 – 6 days of the week depending on your fitness level, and cardio is typically still included 3-4 days of the week at minimal levels for heart and lung conditioning.
8. **Avoid continuing with higher volumes of training and try to "out-train" pour nutrition choices.** It won't work. It will backfire every time. And you will over-train and be exhausted and more prone to injury.
9. **Keep things simple**! Quick and easy works best for busy lifestyles. Continue bringing food with you to work and when out and about. Be intentional when you choose to eat out!

Chapter Review:

1. Review your habits. Both the good ones and the "bad" ones. For each, identify what your cue, ritual and reward is.
2. What healthier habits do you want to develop?
3. What rewards do you perceive you would gain from these new habits? What rewards do you think would be the most motivating for you?
4. What are some places or situations that you could practice your new healthy habits and strengthen willpower?
5. What does sustainability mean to you? Does your definition of sustainable line up with the health and fitness outcomes that you want to achieve and keep in your body? If not, are you willing to change your definition?

Chapter 6.

Your New Normal:

And How to Create It

The ONLY way to get to a healthy place and STAY there, (because staying there is the hard part) will be claiming "Healthy and Fit" as part of your IDENTITY.

Healthy choices are a part of WHO you are and WHAT you do. When you make that a part of your DNA, then no matter what life throws at you, you still make healthy choices as best you can because it is your go-to.

When healthy choices are an external thing. When instead of committing to a healthy lifestyle, you decide to go on a "diet", or cut out a food group for 30 days. It's something you'll try for a little while, but you're not embracing this as part of your new "Normal".

It's something you're DOING, instead of someone new that you are BECOMING.

You may reap some short term rewards. But they will be lost when your old identity remains the same, and you divert back to the old habits.

You know all the benefits we have discussed? These happen as a result of a long term commitment, not a short cut, quick fix or temporary change. This is a major reason many people who lose weight, do not keep it off for the long term.

When you commit to a new IDENTITY, you intentionally start shifting the self-talk and tell yourself that you ARE a fit and healthy person. If you have thoughts that are contrary to that, you do the work to intentionally change them.

This does NOT mean perfection. It doesn't mean that every meal is perfect, or you never have a cocktail or cookie again. In a healthy balanced lifestyle there is room for these things too.

What it means is the majority of your choices are healthy ones, because you enjoy the benefits of healthy living so much that you want to make those choices.

If you get off track, then you get back on. If an uncontrollable comes up and things don't go just the way you were hoping, then you persist through them and make the best choices you can. Being fit and healthy is just a part of you. Period.

Action Step #1 – Debunk Labeling Lies.

When you begin a transformation, one of the first things that you learn is how to read a label. You need to know how to look at the food package, and read what is on the inside. With food, it's pretty accurate as these things are governed by the FDA. However, the supplement industry is an entirely different story.

Since supplements aren't governed by the FDA, there is a massive issue with LABELING LIES. Meaning that it will say one thing on the bottle, but if you actually tested the product, the ingredients on the inside would not match what it says on the outside.[8]

[8] There are some EXCELLENT supplements out there which produce products

What is on the inside is "LESS THAN" what it says on the outside.

You may have this same problem. But in REVERSE! When you allow toxic thoughts, negative self-talk, fears and limiting beliefs to become a part of your LABEL you are LYING on your label. When you say you are "LESS THAN" when you are truly "MORE THAN", that is not truth!

When you put a label on yourself, you use the words "I am".

If you are saying things like "I am dumb." "I am fat." "I am too old." "I am too busy." "I am depressed." "I am a failure." "I am not good enough," then you are lying on your own label. These things do NOT match up with what is on the inside. They do not match up with the truth of what is IN you, that you are capable of. As you create your new normal, you must be careful and intentional about what you put after those two little words: I AM.

Action Step #2 - Create a Healthy Environment.

Our environment has a big impact on our choices.

If you are committed to being a healthy person, that means you need to make healthy choices. That will be much easier to do if you create a healthy environment to live and work in.

The top 3 areas to create healthy spaces for yourself are:

Your Home.

---

with honesty and integrity. Magnum Nutraceuticals is the brand I recommend.

1. **Go through your closets and get rid of foods that would cause temptation for you**. If they are already opened, throw them away and then take the trash out of the house. Don't try finishing them up, they aren't going to serve you or your goals. If they are unopened and non-perishable, pack them up and donate them to a food bank or homeless shelter. If foods that aren't good choices for you, are not in the house, you are far less likely to go out and get them in a moment of weakness!
2. **Fill your house with healthy foods to eat**. Your healthy choices start in your shopping cart at the store. Stick with whole foods for the most part.
3. **Keep treats for the kids or spouse in a separate space.** If you have kids (or a spouse that doesn't share your healthy eating habits), and need to have special treats for them, set up a cabinet or shelf that is just for them. Keep in mind, the earlier in life that kids start eating healthy, the better. Kids will mimic behaviors they see at home. Setting a healthy example at home, can set them up for a healthier future.

Your Work:

1. **Talk to your boss**. If you are in an unhealthy work environment (unhealthy treats always around etc.) talk to your boss or manager about bringing in healthy foods instead of unhealthy. Productivity levels in the workplace will increase if people aren't laden with high sugar and processed foods during the day. If you have a work space, keep it free of temptation and have healthy meals or snacks available. If YOU are the boss, change the culture at your workplace by providing healthy food and drink options for your employees! Set the example.

2. **Bring your own food.** Just because there is "free" food at work doesn't mean you have to eat it. Even if it's free of charge, there is a cost when you fill your body with foods that don't make you feel well, don't get you closer to your goals, and slow your brain productivity down.
3. **Pack up a cooler with quick and easy meals that don't take a lot of time to eat**. Pack an extra meal or two in case you have long work hours or something unexpected comes up.
4. **Avoid temptation**. If you have an issue seeing food and not consuming it, while you are working on the mental shifts to overcome that, avoid areas of the workplace where you know temptations will be, as much as possible. Get rid of any hidden treats at your desk.
5. **Bring water!** Avoid consuming soda or diet soda, drink fresh water throughout the day. It will keep you hydrated and energized.

Your Car:

1. **Change your route**. If you are a fast food junkie and need to break the habit, but drive by your favorite food joint on a regular basis, you may want to consider taking an alternate route until new habits are established.
2. **Get rid of any hidden treats that are kept in the car**. A common hidden behavior of those who struggle with living a healthy lifestyle is eating while in the car when others aren't watching. Don't put the temptation there to begin with!
3. **Pack your meals**. Pack up your cooler with all your meals and foods and take it in the car with you. That

way you will have what you need, when you need it, even when you're away from home.

4. **Listen to empowering music or podcasts**. Car time is a great time to listen to empowering podcasts or speakers who will aid you in building mental strength!

These are the three environments that we spend the most time in. Take time to intentionally make sure they are healthy and will set you up for success.

Action Step #3 - Eliminate Negatives (as much as possible).

When you're creating a healthy new identity, it may mean that you need to eliminate negatives from your life. That may be people, places, or things.

If there are people who do not support your goals or want to sabotage you, you may need to reduce or eliminate time spent with them.

Perhaps you have a friend who puts you down because you are making healthy lifestyle changes, or who pressures you to make unhealthy choices in order to fit in.

If it's a close friend, have a talk with them about how this makes you feel. If they continue to do it, then limit the time spent with them or perhaps even stop spending time with them altogether.

The people that you surround yourself with will have an impact on you! If you continue listening to people who tell you that you won't be a success, or who don't want you to be a success, they will drag you down.

This is of course a sad thing, but one thing to remember is that people are a part of your life for either a specific reason, or a specific season, or for a lifetime. (T.D. Jake's has an amazing speech on this!). If they are just for a season, and that season is through, then appreciate it for what it was. But also know that there are many new people out there, who are new potential friends, who WILL support your dreams and goals and push you to success.

Places that are negative environments may or may not be avoidable. If the negative place is a bar or club, those are easy to avoid. But if it's your workplace, then saying "don't go there" may not be so easy! If there are particular people at your workplace who drag you down, if it's possible to limit contact with them, then do it. If they are people who love to engage in conflict, don't engage.

What about negative habits? If you smoke, do drugs or consume too much alcohol, then these habits don't align with being a fit and healthy person. Do the work to let go of these crutches! If you're able to eliminate them cold turkey, then great. If not, then take advantage of the products available for smoking cessation, or if alcoholism is a problem, get in to an AA group near you as soon as possible. There is help and there is hope.

If you are in a negative work environment, are there other options you can pursue? If not, then the change needs to come from within you, and that means working on responses and reactions to those around you. Even in a workplace that used to drag you down, you can do the internal work that will allow you to ignore negative comments and not let them in. You can shift your perspective. When you look at naysayers, rather than giving them power over your emotions, feel sorry that they have the need to try to bring you down, so that they can feel better!

Family, or specifically a spouse, makes things tricky! You aren't going to just "eliminate" these people. If you are in a relationship that you have made a lifetime commitment to, then that is a big deal and needs to be taken seriously.

Sit and ask them if they will be a supporter or a saboteur? Do they want to see you achieve your goals? When you ask these questions, the answers (or lack of an answer) will reveal the level of influence you can allow this person to have on your life and your healthy choices.

When it's a spouse or family member in the same house, you will likely still have interaction with them on a regular basis. Keep open lines of communication and let them know how important your goals are to you.

Ultimately, regardless of the people in your life. Just know that YOU and only YOU have the power and responsibility for your choices. Though support at home makes life easier. It's still up to you, even if you have an unsupportive spouse or family.

Don't be afraid to LET GO of the negatives so you can TAKE HOLD of your BEST Life!

Chapter Review:

1. Are there any "labeling lies" that you have claimed for yourself that need to change? What do you say after "I am"? Does it line up with what you want your life to look like?
2. How are you identifying yourself? As a fit and healthy person or something else?
3. Take notice of your environment. Home, work and in your car. Are there any changes that need to be made so that these spaces where you spend the majority of your time are conducive for achieving your goals?
4. Are there negatives that you need to eliminate from your life? Think about people, places or things that are holding you back from success. How can you remove or reduce their influence?
5. Do you have family support? If not, can you have a serious conversation to work towards improving the support you're receiving at home?

Chapter 7.

Confrontation:

Digging in to your How and Why

The final mental secret is the big one. The true game changer.

Most people don't like confrontation. But for many, it's going to be necessary to get to a fully healthy and healed place. Working on changing thoughts and developing habits isn't going to be enough if you have a deep root issue that needs to be addressed first.

Throughout this book, we've covered many ways to rethink fat loss. But we have to dig even deeper to discover why there is such a disparity between people who lose weight and keep it off, and those who lose the weight and gain it back.

For change to last a lifetime, you may need to do some HARD work mentally and emotionally (and physically too!).

As you establish the mental shifts we've discussed, you also need to confront your own "how" and "why". Confronting your own truth can be downright scary.

How did you get to an unhealthy and unhappy place to begin with?

This is self-examination. It's gathering information.

This is not about shaming yourself or beating yourself up for past choices. That needs to be clear. This is about making an observation and looking at the path, choices and circumstances that led to your current state.

Perhaps it was just too many social outings, or the busyness of life which caused healthy eating to get off track. Kids, jobs or travel resulted in a lack of preparation so you found yourself relying on fast food for fuel, and didn't prioritize time for exercise.

Or perhaps the "how" is deeper. Maybe your battle is with food addiction, compulsive overeating, emotional eating as a means of coping with sadness, loneliness, stress or even depression. Food is being used (unsuccessfully) to fill a void in life.

Once you have your "how", you have to confront the "why."

This is where things can get uncomfortable.

The WHY is the root. And if the root isn't dug up, then it will continue to grow and eventually resurface. Maybe not right away, but in time, it will sprout back up.

Confronting the "why" goes beyond looking at the thought patterns that have evolved. It digs into what happened in your life for those patterns to take root to begin with.

Is your "why" hard to look at? Or is it easy for you?

Your why may be as simple as not having healthy role models while growing up, or not having good education in regards to what a healthy lifestyle looks like.

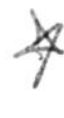

The why may be that you were a former athlete, and once your sport was through you didn't implement activity and healthy eating into your lifestyle.

Maybe you got a job that took all your time and attention, or maybe you decided to build a family and devoted yourself entirely to raising your children and neglected your own health.

For some, it may be an unexpected curveball or trauma that threw you into a tailspin. The loss of a loved one, death of a child, a disease or illness of yourself or a family member, or perhaps divorce or a financial distress.

Maybe you found out your spouse was cheating on you, or were verbally demoralized by a parent, which led you to believe that you are unworthy of love. Since loving yourself is a main reason to take care of your health and body, if you feel unlovable that can lead to neglecting the amazing gift you've been given.

Sadly, the root of "why" for many people is abuse. This could be mental, verbal, emotional, sexual or physical abuse from a parent or partner or other individual earlier in life.

Childhood sexual abuse impacts as many as one in five females and one in six males.[9] This abuse leaves deep hurt, trauma and scars that can be extremely painful to look at. But if the pain is hidden away and not dealt with, it can, and likely will manifest in unhealthy ways.

---

[9] If you are a victim of sexual assault or childhood sexual abuse please visit www.rainn.org to find local resources to help and support you.

I've been heartbroken when hearing from clients who were sexually abused, and used food and weight gain as a way to make their body undesirable so that they would feel safe.

Though they didn't like living in an unhealthy body, they continually reverted back to eating and the weight gain as a way to avoid unwanted attention. It was their defense against getting hurt again. It was their coping mechanism for dealing with the pain and trauma that was so hard and ugly to face.

These are deep issues. If your "why" is rooted in this way, then know that there is help out there for you. There is work that will need to be done, but there is freedom in doing it.

My advice would be to get in to see a licensed counselor or therapist on a regular basis, for as long as needed, as you sort through pain and emotions and behaviors.

Do the work. Dig in. Dive deep.

Everyone has a story. Everyone has "stuff" to deal with. Some more than others. Get into your stuff, don't shy away from it.

In fact, do the work, no matter how hard it is, and then take it a step further and help others who are going through what you have survived.

Many people need help. Your healing, your health, may be the key to someone else's freedom from the bondage of a painful and traumatic past.

Here are the steps to confrontation:

1. **Map out "how" you got to an unhealthy place**. The place where you desire change.

2. **Do not shame or guilt yourself for any past behaviors.** Observe how things came to be from an inquisitive mindset.
3. **Dig deeper and ask the hard "why"**. What is the root of unhealthy mindsets or behaviors to begin with?
4. **If the "why" includes trauma or abuse, please get in to see a licensed counselor or therapist who can help you sort through pain and emotions and work to a place of healing.**
5. **DIG IN**. No matter how long it takes, keep digging and if healing or forgiveness needs to take place, then do the work to get there. Don't let the past hold you back from your best, healthiest future.

Chapter Review:

1. How did you get where you are today?
2. Why is your current situation what it is? Do you know the root?
3. Have you gone through any type of abuse, whether emotional, mental, physical or sexual that is a part of your why?
4. If yes to the above. Have you sought out help? Are you willing to speak counselor to help you navigate trauma or abuse that you have gone through?

If you have gone through trauma or abuse, PLEASE seek out and ask for the help that you need. There are people (myself included!) who want to see you healed and whole and able to live your life to the fullest. There are a LOT of people CARE about what you have gone through and want to help. If you would like my help finding a counseling resource in your area, please write to me at** diana.chaloux@yahoo.com **.

Bonus Section 1.

ARE YOU READY?

Now you know the top seven mental secrets for rethinking fat loss. What do you think?

Are you ready for change?

Don't jump to "yes" right away. Take your time and consider.

When you're SURE that the answer to this question is yes, then it's time to begin your journey.

Saying yes means that you're not just thinking about making change, you're ready to take action. There have been a lot of action tips throughout this book, and those are your first steps. Maybe you don't take ALL the actions in one day, but you're ready to take at least one.

Readiness to change is so important. At Hitch Fit, we always ask that a client be truly ready for change. Starting before you're ready is frustrating. Because progress, success and sustainability will all take action. Repeated action. It's not "one and done" when it comes to your health and fitness. Frustration and discouragement ensue when no progress is made, and that often leads to quitting. You just end up STUCK at the starting gate!

Be ready. Don't think it's going to be perfect. Just be ready to dig in and do the work and be persistent. Run the race that is set before you!

1. **Be Committed not just "Interested".**

Once you know you're ready, be committed.

There are many people who "want" to get in shape, have a lot of energy, like how they look and feel, get off medication, have higher self-esteem and strength.

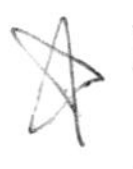

But wanting it is NOT enough.

Nearly everyone wants it! That's why weight loss is a multi-billion dollar industry (with an incredibly high failure rate!)

There is a big difference between wanting change, and wanting it ENOUGH, with specific goals and motivation, to actually take the action steps to be successful! The key to the "want" becoming a reality, lies completely in the ACTION phase. This is where most people fall short.

Those who are just "interested" in change or improvements want the end result, but are not willing to do the work and take the actions to make it happen.

Those who are "committed" want the end result and are READY to take the actions necessary for success.

Are you interested? Or are you committed?

2. **Be Consistent and Persistent**

Consistency is key. You have to be consistent with your choices if you want to succeed. Just doing something for a week or a month isn't going to lead to long term goal achievement. If you want success in any aspect of your life to be reached and then sustained, you must stay consistent with the choices and actions that made you successful to begin with!

You also need to be persistent.

Your journey will have lots of ups and downs! Life throws a lot of things in our way. The way to be successful for the long term, is by persisting around, over or through any obstacles that come up along the way.

3. **SHOW UP (Even when you don't feel like it).**

Do you feel like doing your job every day?

Do you wake up EVERY day and you can't wait to working?

Can't wait to go to that meeting, can't wait to prepare that presentation, can't wait to serve tables, can't wait to fire that employee? Can't wait to _____ (you can fill in the blanks with whatever your daily duties happen to be!).

Most people, if they are being honest, don't feel like working EVERY day. I mean, I LOVE what I do. I love the chance to help people transform their lives. It is an incredible feeling. But there are days when I don't "feel" like going to the gym, or I don't "feel" like working on websites or writing back to the never ending emails in my inbox.

But guess what, if I want to be successful. I have to SHOW UP even on the days that I don't feel like it.

Here's another shocker! I don't ALWAYS feel like working out or making a healthy eating choice! (Say what?) Nope! I'm not a robot that never has days where I'm tired or worn out, or days where I just don't feel like eating well.

BUT I have to SHOW UP in my life, and do the things that need to be done that keep me where I want to be. And that means showing up even when I don't feel like it.

If you don't go to work because you don't "feel" like it, what would happen? Well you may be fired and lose your job, or if you are a business owner your company may go out of business.

Your physical health and fitness is the same!

You will have days that you don't feel like getting up, or getting that work out in, or making the healthy choice. But you've got to SHOW UP. That may mean just getting yourself to the gym (sometimes the hardest part is just getting started!). Showing up may mean making the healthy choice at a restaurant instead of something that you know will make you feel poorly later.

You show up so that your life and choices line up with the goals that are worth it to you to work for.

It's time for your answer.

Are you READY?

Bonus Section 2.

25 Tips to Maintain Motivation

Motivation is a word we hear every day! When a person ceases to make the choices necessary to reach a goal they claim to have, one of the most common excuses for lack of adherence is "loss of motivation".

Motivation is a driving force that either comes from within you, or from an external pressure that compels you to make the necessary choices and take the actions that enable you to achieve the goal at hand.

To avoid falling off the wagon, or losing your drive, here are 25 tips to help you maintain your motivation!

1. **Develop a positive attitude**: Negativity towards what is necessary to achieve what you want in life will only set you up for failure. Stay focused on the positive, write down the positives that are in your life right now, and all the wonderful things that you will achieve, feel and see happen in your life when you make the right choices day in and day out. Your attitude towards anything in life is completely under your control, take charge of that power and you can see the upside of any situation.

2. **Identify your obstacles:** You may have made excuses for years as to why you don't possess the power and

responsibility to make the choices necessary to achieve your goals. Own up to the excuses and identify them as obstacles that you can now overcome. Early on, identify the obstacles that are going to pop up along the way, and come up with strategies that you will incorporate to get around them when they occur.

3. **Find an exercise mode that you enjoy**: There are plenty of ways that you can train in order to achieve your fitness goals. Try new things and find methods that you enjoy. Waking up and dreading what you have to do will usually result in skipping your workout. Whether it's strength training in the gym, playing your favorite sport or heading out for a hike or bike ride, figure out what is going to energize you and that you will adhere to.

4. **Exercise with a friend**: This is a great way to stay accountable. If you are more motivated knowing that someone is at the gym or on the hiking trail waiting for you, then finding a workout buddy will be a great way for you to stay on track. Working out with a loved one or a friend can be rewarding in many ways. This can boost your relationship as you become closer and healthier together! Many people feel nervous when going to a new gym so signing up with a friend can eliminate much of that fear!

5. **Set realistic goals:** Goal setting is crucial, much like your job you will have goals, quotas or projections that you want to meet. Set goals that are attainable for you,

set short term goals and long term goals. Do not set goals that are out of reach as that will set you up for disappointment. For example, don't shoot to lose 40 pounds in a month, you want to set goals that are going to get you on a healthy track and keep you on that track for the rest of your life.

6. **Compete**: Competing is a great way to push yourself to new levels, it adds a level of excitement to attaining your goals, and knowing that those who you are competing against may be out there working harder than you, or that slacking on your training will prevent you from finishing a race or winning an ultimate prize, you will find you are much more motivated to stay on track.

7. **Educate:** The more educated you are about how your body works, and about how nutrition affects and changes your body, the easier it will be for you to make good choices about your own personal health and fitness. Ignorance is bliss, until it leads to health issues, self-esteem issues, and/or disappointment in what you have allowed your body to become. The information you need to achieve your goals is out there, it's just up to you to seek it out.

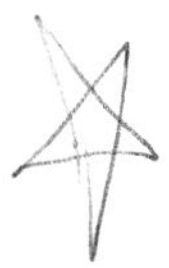

8. **Move:** The only way you are going to add that muscle, drop body fat and transform your physique is to MOVE. If an hour of exercise seems daunting at first, just get moving for 5 minutes, you will find that once you get your body in action it is much easier to keep it going.

9. **Change your scenery**: Revamp your workouts with a change of scenery. Go to a different gym to switch things up or take your training outside.

10. **Try something new:** A consistent workout routine as part of your day to day life is absolutely beneficial, but to avoid boredom don't be afraid to try something new. Maybe you've always wanted to try Pilates, or learn karate or try out that cool kickboxing class. Mix things up and keep them fresh by branching out and trying something you've always wanted to.

11. **Listen to music**: Studies show that music elevates your mood and can enhance your workouts. Having your favorite beats playing while you are strength training or doing cardio can help you keep going even when you are tired. If you are slowing down or thinking of prematurely quitting, kick on one of your favorite songs and you will get a surge of rejuvenation.

12. **Track your measurements and workouts**: When you first set out to achieve your goals, be sure to know where you are starting from so that you will know how much progress you have made over the course of time. Track your stats and measurements and track your workouts. It's exciting to see when you could only do 4 push-ups on day one and 12 weeks later you can do 50! If you don't track your progress you will not know how far you have come. If you are having a tough day, a great way to get reenergized is by checking your stats and

seeing positive progress in the right direction, letting you know that your hard work is paying off.

13. **Take Pictures**: When you start out on a fitness journey, it is highly likely that you will hate your starting point, regardless of what that might be. The majority of people are motivated to visually look better, so seeing the condition of their current physique can be difficult. Nevertheless this is a critical piece of the puzzle, to actually SEE the changes in your body instead of just FEEL them is very powerful. Take pictures every 2-4 weeks to see the change in your body. Post your pictures someplace that you can see them every day so that you will remember why you are making the right choices day in and day out.

14. **Journal your nutrition**: When you are working towards attaining a fitness or health goal, 80% of your success is going to depend on the eating choices that you are making on a day to day basis. Stay on track and motivated by writing down all that you eat in a given day, this will also help you avoid mindlessly snacking or going over the amount of calories that you should be taking in per day.

15. **Reward yourself**: The internal rewards of achieving a fitness goal are great, however giving yourself an external reward can increase your motivation even further. A couple ideas to positively reinforce without having a fitness setback are purchasing a new pair of

running shoes or workout clothes, or enjoying some pampering at the spa.

16. **Schedule your workouts**: We all have extremely busy lives. Our time is consumed by jobs, families and any number of activities which will easily pull our attention away from taking work out time for ourselves. Putting your health and fitness on the back burner just sets you up for long term health issues and unhappiness. Your fitness IS important, so take the time to schedule your workouts into your day. Treat it as an important appointment that you can't miss, and make sure you get it done!

17. **Find YOUR right time**: You may be a morning person or perhaps you are an evening person. Regardless of which time of day you find yourself most energized, you can achieve your goals. Plan your training schedule accordingly so that you hit your workout of choice at the time when you feel strongest and most eager to exercise.

18. **Eliminate negatives**: Cutting negative people, places and circumstances out of your life will open you up for more positives. To the best of your ability, avoid negative people who would put you down, negative places that cause you to fall off track or put you in a bad mood, and negative circumstances that can lead you to emotional stress and poor choice making. Cutting all negatives in your life out may not be an option, but do your best to eliminate as many of them as possible.

19. **Get creative in the kitchen**: Eating healthy is crucial to your fitness success, and good foods can taste great. The only way you are going to enjoy eating healthy for a lifetime is if you find foods that you enjoy eating on a daily basis. Find ways of preparing your foods that please your palate. You've got options including but not limited to, grilling, baking or steaming. Hit up the spices aisle at your local grocery store and find some new ways to flavor your meats and veggies, there are loads of options out there.

20. **Be prepared:** Preparation is the key to your success. If you are consistently unprepared, meaning you don't have the right foods available at the right times, or you forgot your gym clothes, then you can easily lose your motivation and fall off track. Schedule the time on weekends or during your "down" times to cook your foods and having them ready to go when you need them. Tupperware to store these items in your fridge or freezer as well as a small cooler so you can take your food with you to work or out running errands will help you stay on track.

21. **Talk to your family:** Family support can be one of the make or break aspects to achieving your fitness goals. A home filled with naysayers is difficult to avoid, so it's important that early on in your journey you sit them down, have a heart to heart explaining your goals and why they are important to you. Explain that you need their support in order to achieve them. If this doesn't

work, you CAN still achieve your goals, it will just be a matter of tapping into a deeper level of inner strength.

22. **Join an online fitness community**: When you are working towards a fitness goal, it helps when you know there are others out there working towards similar aspirations and struggling with similar obstacles. Having an online support team can be especially important if you are lacking encouragement at home.

23. **Find a great personal trainer**: Having a quality trainer to motivate you and guide you can be the piece of the puzzle that will get you to your goals. A good trainer will help you set goals; and guide you on the lifestyle, eating and exercise choices that will get you there. Knowing that you have a trainer to teach you, push you, hold you accountable and keep you on track, can help you get to your goals if it is within your budget. There are also online training programs (such as what we offer at Hitch Fit www.hitchfit.com) which enable you to virtually work with a personal trainer at a fraction of the cost of one on one. If budget is an issue, or you don't have a qualified trainer close to you, then online may be the best option for you.

24. **Practice positive affirmations:** Belief in yourself is critical to your success. You may doubt your ability and find yourself engaging in negative self-talk. If that is the case then you must begin positive affirmations on a daily basis. When positively affirming be sure that you

use present tense such as "I am" rather than "I will". Come up with a list of 5-10 positive affirmations about yourself and repeat them on a daily basis. Over time these positive thoughts will become engrained in your mind and will be a natural part of how you think of yourself. Even if you already have a positive though process, affirmations can make your mind even more powerful over your ability to succeed at your goals.

25. **Create habits and focus on lifestyle**: When it comes to weight loss, you don't want to just lose weight for a short period of time only to gain it all back. Look at your new healthy eating and exercise choices as your new powerful, positive and healthy lifestyle, not as something you are just doing briefly. Focus on creating new habits and embracing a new way of living. Visualize making these healthy choices not just today and tomorrow, but picture yourself in one year, five years or ten years making these same choices and still living the life that imagine for yourself.

Hitch Fit Library

Buy all the Hitch Fit Books!
Titles available on Amazon.com

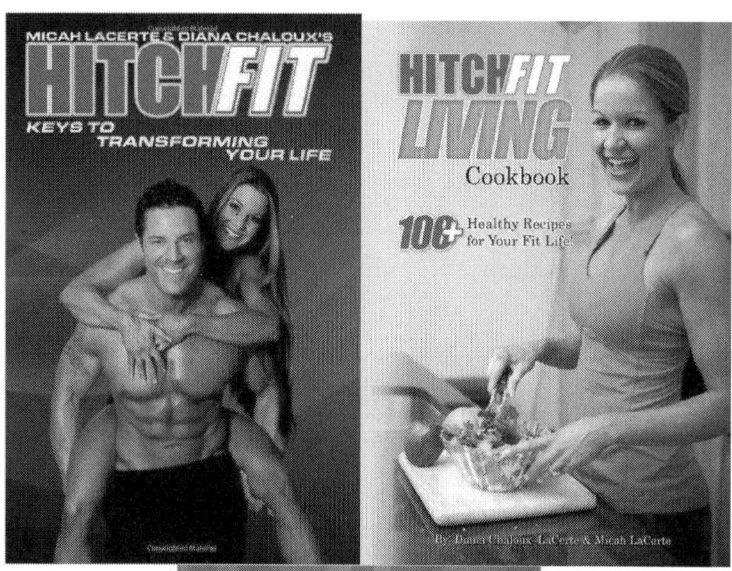

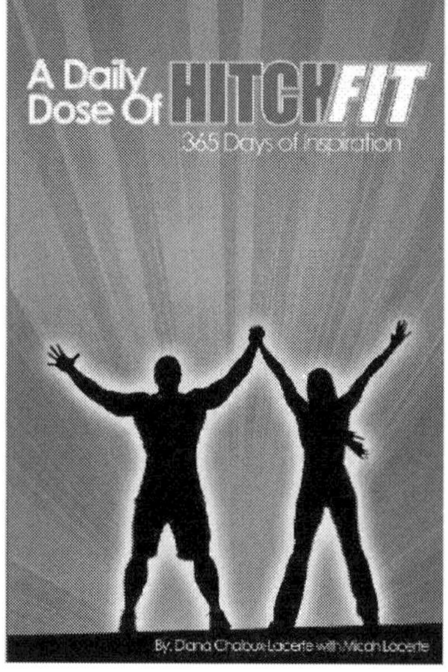

About the Author

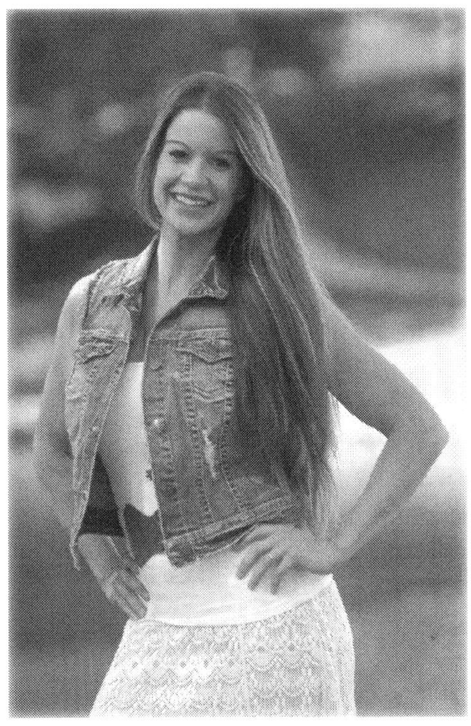

Diana Chaloux – LaCerte is an author, entrepreneur, co-founder and co-owner of Hitch Fit Gym and Hitch Fit Online Personal Training, based in Kansas City, MO. She is a health and fitness expert, and world champion fitness athlete, with a passion for leading others to strength in mind, body and spirit. Diana and husband and Hitch Fit co-owner Micah reside in Kansas City and have been married since 2011. Write to her at diana.chaloux@yahoo.com . Visit www.Hitchfit.com for online coaching options.

Ready to Transform with Hitch Fit?

Thank you for reading *Rethinking Fat Loss*! If you are ready to transform your life, and commit to being a fit and healthy person, then we would love to help you on that journey. Hitch Fit has been transforming lives since 2009. Micah and Diana LaCerte offer online personal training to clients globally, and also own and operate one on one personal training gyms in the Kansas City area. Check out program options, that include nutrition, training and online support at www.HitchFit.com .

Websites:
www.HitchFit.com
www.HitchFitGym.com

Instagram:
@DianaChaloux
@MicahLaCerte
@HitchFit
@HitchFitGym

Facebook:
www.facebook.com/dianachaloux
www.facebook.com/micahlacerte
www.facebook.com/hitchfit

Youtube:
www.youtube.com/hitchfit
www.youtube.com/dianachaloux
www.youtube.com/micahlacerte

Linkedin:
www.linkedin.com/in/dianachaloux/
www.linkedin.com/in/hitchfit/

Made in the USA
Monee, IL
10 August 2021

75385816R00067